Instrumentation and Applications of Hyphenated Techniques

Instrumentation and Applications of Hyphenated Techniques

Adikay Sreedevi
M.Pharm, Ph.D

Professor
Institute of Pharmaceutical Technology,
Sri Padmavati Mahila Visvavidyalayam
Tirupati – 517502

Kaveripakam Sai Sruthi
M.Pharm, Ph.D

Assistant Professor (C)
Institute of Pharmaceutical Technology,
Sri Padmavati Mahila Visvavidyalayam
Tirupati - 517502

Kakarla Sushmitha
B.Pharm, (M. Pharm)

Institute of Pharmaceutical Technology,
Sri Padmavati Mahila Visvavidyalayam
Tirupati - 517502

Gottipalli Sri Jaswanthi
B.Pharm, (M.Pharm)

Institute of Pharmaceutical Technology,
Sri Padmavati Mahila Visvavidyalayam
Tirupati - 517502

PharmaMed Press
An imprint of BSP Books Pvt. Ltd
4-4-309/316, Giriraj Lane,
Sultan Bazar, Hyderabad - 500 095.

Instrumentation and Applications of Hyphenated Techniques
***by* Adikay Sreedevi, Kakarla Sushmitha, Gottipalli Sri Jaswanthi and Kaveripakam Sai Sruthi**

Published by:

Pharma Med PRESS
An Imprint of
BSP Books Pvt. Ltd.

PharmaMed Press

An imprint of BSP Books Pvt. Ltd.
4-4-309/316, Giriraj Lane, Sultan Bazar, Hyderabad - 500 095.
Phone: 040-23445688; Fax: 91+40-23445611
e-mail: info@pharmamedpress.com
www.pharmamedpress.com/pharmamedpress.net

ISBN: 978-93-48734-42-6 (Hardback)

Preface

In this dynamic realm of Pharmaceutical sciences, the subject of this book's exploration is "Instrumentation & Applications of Hyphenated Techniques". This textbook is primarily intended for emphasizing the fundamental concepts in the core area of various hyphenated analytical techniques. This book includes chapters on various hyphenated techniques such as GC-MS, LC-MS, LC-NMR, LC-IR etc. Each chapter demystifies the principle, instrumentation and applications of these techniques. This work serves as a theoretical guide that highlights the practical applications of these techniques, bridging the gap between academics and industry. With the expertise of authors readers will gain invaluable insights into various hyphenated analytical approaches. Prioritizing the development of vital competencies, this book serves as a beacon for students seeking to excel in the turbulent field of analytical chemistry. With current hyphenation, the notions written are more beneficial to all pharmacy professionals in teaching and research in any area of the analytical world.

- Authors

Contents

CHAPTER 1

Introduction to Analytical Chemistry

Introduction

One of the most important branches of chemistry is analytical chemistry, which deals with the identification, separation, and quantification of the relative concentrations of various elements in a sample. It is focused on providing answers to inquiries on both the quantitative and qualitative features of matter and its chemical characterization. The Big Data Era has entwined itself more and more with analytical chemistry over the course of the last 20 years, challenging long-held theories and bringing about paradigm changes within the field.

A key scientific field that supplies data to other fields including materials science, nanotechnologies, biological and physiological sciences, and engineering is analytical chemistry. But in the previous 20 years, it has seen a "metamorphosis" that calls for a reconsideration of its foundations, place in science, educational components, methods, regulations, and criteria.

The norms, ideals, and definitions associated with analytical science and chemical analysis need to be rethought in light of the current state of uncertainty in these fields and the need to move past antiquated conceptions. It is important to examine how definitions, regulations, processes, techniques, and procedures changed from the 1960s onward to meet modern demands because they are products of their respective eras. Addressing misconceptions and expectations about analytical chemistry can enhance its significance and application in modern science and technology.

Analytical chemistry: how it evolved

With the field entering the Big Science Era, analytical chemistry has seen tremendous growth since the 1960s. Analytical techniques cantered around the relationship of particles and radiation have been introduced in this age, spanning from hard X-rays to the terahertz domain. Because it makes it possible to link the in situ chemical makeup of smaller study objects to the delicate interaction of radiation with matter, spectrometer has grown into an indispensable characterization tool across multiple scientific and industrial areas. Significant enhancements in particularity, sensitivity, spatial discrimination, and analysis speed have been made possible by a variety of mass spectrometry and spectroscopy techniques, using fully automated analytical equipment.

The resulting comprehensive suite of analytical techniques is a powerful force in scientific advancement, but it must now tackle issues of ever-increasing complexity using techniques that call for ever-faster, repetitive measurements of an ever-wider range of fundamental and intricate molecular substances and structural configurations. Over the past fifty years, advancements in electronic devices, technological innovations, laboratory equipment firms, smaller and nanotechnologies and generalized scientific advances in biological sciences, chemistry, and physics have all contributed to the growth of analytical chemistry. These developments have been driven by tools and concepts.

Analytical chemistry definition: In the field of analytical chemistry, chemicals are isolated, identified, and quantified employing both conventional and advanced techniques and equipment from science. It entails the separation between chemical elements, free radicals, or functional groups. Quantitative evaluation provides statistical data about the relative quantities of species, whereas qualitative analysis provides information about the nature of an atomic in nature, molecular, or biomolecular species. The science of gathering, analyzing, and disseminating data on the make-up and arrangement of matter allows scientists to define and quantify matter. This is known as analytical chemistry.

Role of analytical chemistry: The critical science of analytical chemistry is concerned with producing new information to enhance chemical evaluation in response to growing or novel needs. It is crucial in many different fields of study, including food production, medical diagnostics, controlling processes, environmental monitoring, and forensic surveys. Crucial choices about medical care, environmental contamination thresholds, and soil remediation could not be made without analytical chemistry. Over time, the main objective in analytical chemistry has changed from analyzing elements and speciation towards instrument development, with the development process being driven by instrument makers.

Due to pressing biological demands, mass spectrometry is now a helpful instrument for chemists, pharmacologists, doctors, and biologists. Increased efforts in analytical chemistry and general chemistry are needed for sustainable development operations in the chemical sector. Analytical chemistry frequently supports methodological and experimental design,

method encouragement monitoring of quality, multivariate analysis of information, and interpretation of outcomes in collaborative initiatives.

Engineers, researchers in biology, medical learners, sociologists, and legislators all take analytical chemistry courses, which continue to be an essential component of undergraduate chemistry education. Out of 16 optional chemistry courses, it comes in third, demonstrating the need for more research and instruction in analytical chemistry.

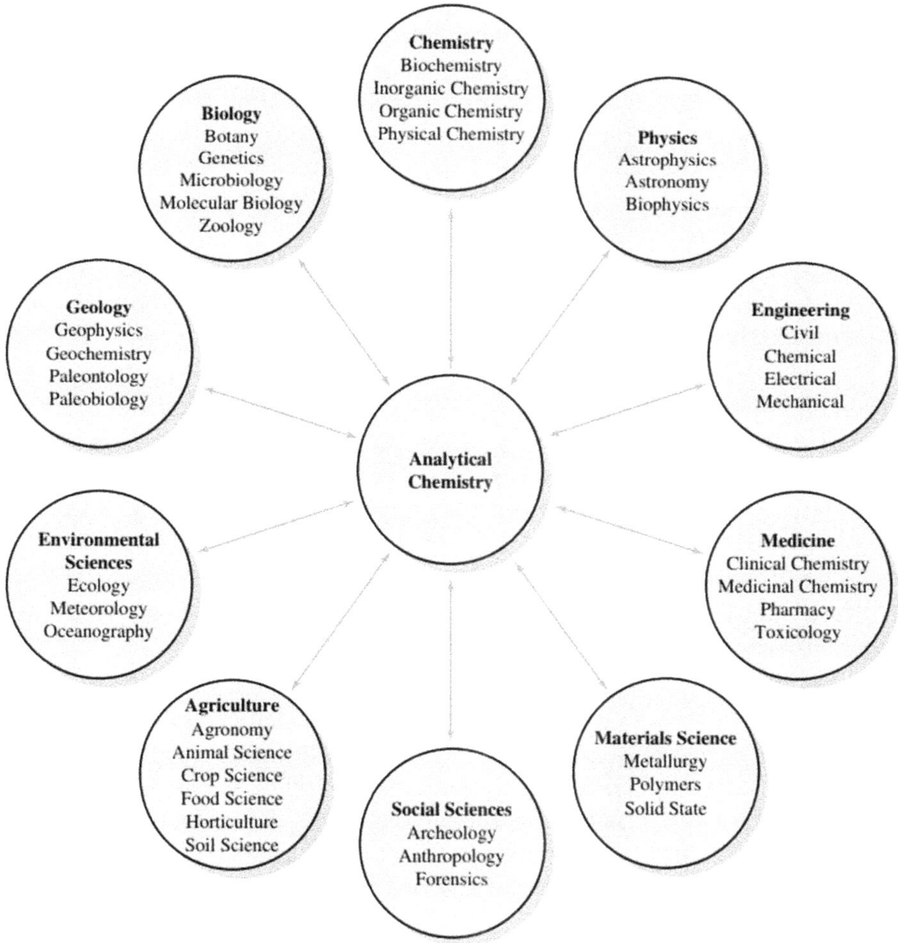

The science of analytical chemistry is essential to the chemical industry for the identification, quantification, and detection of pharmaceuticals and foreign substances in biological material. It assists in identifying contaminants and adulterants as well as assesses if the product is within acceptable levels of contamination. Analytical chemistry is heavily dependent on diagnosis within healthcare technology and research, including blood glucose, urine ketones, and serum cholesterol levels.

Importance of analytical chemistry in various fields: Clinical tests performed in medicine are based on analytical chemistry and are used to assist doctors diagnose illnesses and track patients' progress toward recovery.

Analytical chemistry is used in industry to analyze raw materials and guarantee the quality of completed goods where the chemical makeup is crucial. An analytical chemist develops processes for the analysis of a wide range of items, including paints, fuels, home goods, medications, and more, before they are marketed to consumers. Analytical chemistry techniques are frequently used to test for potential pollutants in order to evaluate the quality of the natural world. Chemical analysis is used to assess the health benefits of food for main components like protein and carbohydrates as well as trace elements like minerals and vitamins. In fact, a food's calories are frequently determined by chemical analysis.

1. **Analytical chemistry is concerned with the analysis of samples, both quantitative and qualitative**

   Quantitative chemistry's primary objective is to perform qualitative and quantitative evaluations of samples. Analytical chemists detect the analyte and calculate its concentration in a given sample using a variety of chemical processes and methods. Simple weighing jobs to complex studies utilizing high-tech equipment like an Ion Chromatograph (IC), Gas Chromatograph (GC), High-Performance Liquid Chromatograph (HPLC), Mass Spectrometer (MS), and others are covered by these procedures.

2. **Both organic and heterogeneous chemistry labs use analytical chemistry**

   Several areas of chemistry are frequently connected to one another and cooperate to address a variety of problems. Evidently, both organic and inorganic chemists utilize analytical chemistry techniques extensively. For instance, analytical chemistry techniques are used by scientists to ascertain sample concentrations and product contents. Additionally, analytical chemistry enables organic chemists to use infrared spectroscopy (IR) to detect functional groups in an existing sample or a freshly generated chemical.

3. **The foundation of instrumental chemistry is basic analytical chemical techniques**

   Based on fundamental analytical chemistry concepts, instrumental biochemistry is a subfield of analytical chemistry. Despite the fact that instrumental chemistry uses even with the mostsophisticated technologies, conducting studies and assessing outcomes still demands an understanding of even the most basic analytical techniques.

4. **Clinical laboratory technicians can analyze individual biological samples with the help of analytical chemistry**

   The biochemical examination of human biological material or bodily fluids is the foundation of clinical chemistry. Analytical chemistry techniques are used to examine your biospecimens when you take a blood, urine, or saliva test. Simple chemical reactions are needed for certain studies, whereas instrumental sample analyses are needed for others. In any event, clinical lab scientists can accurately provide the laboratory test findings that a doctor is looking for through analytical chemistry.

5. **Healthcare workers can recognize and treat illnesses according to analytical chemistry**

   Analytical chemistry not only makes bodily fluid studies possible for clinical lab scientists, but it also aids medical practitioners in diagnosing conditions and suggesting efficient course of therapy. Physicians can make a variety of diagnoses by determining the quantity of hazardous waste or the quantity of nutrients present in bodily fluids. Analytical testing, both quantitative and qualitative, are also essential for developing treatment strategies that take into account the patient's body's various chemical levels.

6. **Analytical chemistry is important in forensic sciences**

   In order to support investigations, forensic science studies and evaluates evidence from crime scenes. It resolves complicated issues using both basic and sophisticated strategies. The fields of analytical science and molecular biology are becoming more important in forensic investigations. Drug analysis, forensic pathology, DNA analysis, and trace evidence investigation are examples of common forensic tests. Blood analysis, DNA fingerprint identification, and criminology-related analysis are all included in forensic analysis. The identification and examination of biological components are aspects of bioanalytical chemistry and analysis.

7. **Pharmaceutical product development involves analytical chemistry techniques**

   Researching, creating, and managing the standard of pharmaceutical goods all depend on analytical chemistry. Through a battery of analytical tests, scientists are able to better assess the safety and efficacy of novel medications. Although HPLC is the main analytical technique utilized in the pharmaceutical sector, other techniques are also commonly employed. Chemists wasn't going have been able to investigate the chemical and physical characteristics of pharmaceuticals without analytical chemistry. Because of this, the development of safe and effective pharmaceutical products depends heavily on analytical chemistry.

8. Analytical chemistry is essential to reducing pollution in the environment

Pollution of the air, water, and land are all considered forms of environmental pollution, and they have a wide range of detrimental effects on our world. Since pollution from industry is the main contributor to climate change, it is critical to monitor and manage the level and composition of pollutants in the environment. And this is where the application of analytical chemistry is made. Analytical chemists assist environmental scientists in assessing the level of pollution in the environment by examining the contents of the air, water, and land. Research on controlling pollution levels and reducing the number of hazardous compounds released into the environment can benefit from this knowledge.

9. The use of analytical chemicals in precise quality-control analysis

Numerous uses for analytical chemistry exist in quality control. We can be confident that the food and water we consume are safe to consume thanks to accurate assessments. Drug effectiveness and purity can also be verified by analytical techniques. Furthermore, it is the duty of environmental analytical chemists to keep an eye on the amount of greenhouse gases that exist in the atmosphere. We might not have been able to utilize effective medications or consume nutritious meals without analytical chemistry.

10. Analytical chemistry is important in agricultural industry

In the field of agriculture, analytical chemistry is essential to maintaining soil fertility, increasing crop output, and improving crop quality. Professionals may use it to detect fungal contaminations, assess soil nutrients and harmful metal levels, and test pesticides. It is applied to tough crop examination, evaluation of water, and soil testing. Assessing soil looks at both organic and inorganic minerals to see if it is suitable for growing crops and for the microbiological environment. Hard water can deposit lime on rich soil, rendering it unsuitable for agriculture. Water testing can assist discover this. Lastly, severe crop testing assesses pollutants and pesticide residues in harvested crops. Plant material is rejected for use by humans if it has a high concentration of insecticide or other waste. All things considered; analytical chemistry is essential to the agronomic industry.

Analytical chemistry

Analytical techniques categorize into:

A. Chemical
B. Instrumental Techniques

Chemical procedures involve basic glassware manipulation and chemical processes, while instrumental approaches use intricate instruments for energy quantification and sample makeup.

Combining chemical and instrumental procedures is often the optimal approach for addressing issues, with advancements in analytical measures largely attributed to general instrumentation breakthroughs.

Benefits of the instrumental approach:

1. Its speedy determination (it may be done in as little as 1/100 of a second).
2. It's possible to utilize little samples.
3. Difficult samples are manageable.
4. There is an increase in sensitivity.
5. Measurements are achieved with reliability.

Benefits of the chemical approach:

1. The processes are basic simplicity.
2. The methods are precise.
3. The techniques typically rely on precise measurements.
4. Often, specialized training is not necessary.
5. The necessary equipment is reasonably priced.

Limitations of chemical approaches:

1. Their lack of specificity.
2. Procedures typically take a lot of time.
3. As quantities decrease, accuracy declines.
4. The lack of adaptability is evident.
5. The chemical atmosphere is important.

Limitations of Instrumental approaches:

1. There must be an initial calibration, or ongoing calibration.
2. The calibration wet chemical technique or reference instrument determines the accuracy and sensitivity.
3. The final accuracy is often 15% or less.
4. Complex equipment has high initial and ongoing costs.

5. There is a restricted concentration range.
6. It often takes a large amount of space.
7. Specialized instruction is required.

A. Classical (Chemical):

Classical analytical techniques rely on chemical reactions for analysis, while instrumental techniques measure an analyte's physical characteristics.

Classical qualitative analysis: In classical qualitative analysis, one or more chemical reagents are added to the analyte, allowing identification through chemical reactions and byproducts. These reagents react selectively with a single class of chemical compounds, producing a unique reaction product, typically colored or vapor or precipitate.

Classical organic qualitative analysis involves chemical interactions between organic molecules' functional groups and reagents, often yielding fragmentary information. To identify the whole molecule, functional group analysis is combined with other measures like densities, melting temperatures, and boiling points. This method can be complex due to the multitude of potential chemical species in the combination.

Classical quantitative analysis: Classical quantitative analysis categorizes into:

I. Gravimetric analysis
II. Volumetric analysis

Analyte and other reagents undergo extensive chemical reactions in both procedures.

I. Gravimetric analysis: The foundation of gravimetry is the capacity to transform the intended component into a pure, measurable form. Precipitation, electrodeposition, and volatilization are methods that can be used for this.

Precipitation of the desired element, filtering, drying, and weighing of the precipitate are the steps involved in producing a pure sample via precipitation.

In electrodeposition, a current is sent *Via* an electrode to isolate the desired ingredient. The quantity of the intended ingredient may be determined by weighing the electrode both before and after the plating operation.

The electrodeposition method and volatilization are comparable in that they both record a weight differential. In this instance, a known stoichiometric reaction breaks down the sample, and one of the products is volatilized. The quantity of vaporized ingredient is shown by the weight

difference between the pre- and post-volatilization states. Generally speaking, weight loss results from a compound's destruction.

II. Volumetric analysis: Titrimetric analysis, also known as volumetric analysis, involves adding a reagent (titrant) to an analyte slowly or stepwise using a burette. The equivalency point, indicated by a color change, is crucial for successful titrimetric studies. A chemical indicator is introduced before the titration to prevent spontaneous color changes. Chemical indicators undergo color changes at or near equivalency points in acid-base, oxidation-reduction, complexation, and precipitation titrations. The titration ends when the amount of titrant matches the indicator color change. When combined with the known titrant concentration, the end point serves as an estimate of the equivalency point and is utilized to determine the amount or concentration of the analyte.

Volumetric titrations come in four kinds, each of which based on a particular kind of reaction.

a. Acid-base titration

b. Oxidation-reduction titration

c. Precipitation titration

d. Complexometric titration

a. Acid-base titration: There is a neutralizing reaction during an acid-base titration. Titration with a suitable standard base solution is used to determine acids, while titration with a suitable standard acid solution is used to determine bases.

An acid-base titration can be carried out in a solvent other than water, and the choice of solvent can often dictate whether the analysis is successful or not.

b. Oxidation-reduction titration: In an oxidation-reduction titration, the titrant and the chemical being evaluated undergo a change in oxidation state.

The titrant and sample must be in stoichiometric amounts and at the proper oxidation state.

c. Precipitation titration: A precipitation titration and the gravimetric technique are comparable. The distinction is that a stoichiometric amount of precipitating agent (the titrant) is supplied and the volume required for the reaction is determined, as opposed to employing an excess of precipitating agent. The precipitating agent solution is a standard solution; thus, it is possible to determine how much of the desired element is present. Precipitation methods generally only work with a limited range of species and have trouble identifying the titration's stoichiometric point in a practical and straightforward manner.

d. **Complexometric titration:** A complex is formed as a result of the reaction that occurs in a complexometric titration, when the titrant is a complexing agent.

   It's not possible to employ every complex-former as a titrant. In actuality, the majority don't fulfill the conditions necessary to be an effective titrant. The last 15 to 20 years have seen the most exploitation of this kind of titration.

   There has to be a way for figuring out the titration's stoichiometric point for all volumetric methods. Depending on the method used—chemical action (color indicators) or instrumental action—the detection system selected should result in a discernible change that happens to coincide with the reaction's stoichiometric point. The equivalence point is the titration's true stoichiometric point, whereas the location that was obtained by experimentation is known as the end point. The titration error distinguishes between the two.

B. Instrumental techniques:

Depending on the characteristic of the analyte that has to be tested, many kinds of instrumental techniques of chemical analysis exist. Numerous techniques are applicable to qualitative as well as quantitative analysis.

The three main types of instrumental techniques are:

I. Spectral
II. Electroanalytical
III. Separative technique

I. Spectral:

Spectral techniques measure the electromagnetic radiation analyte absorbs, scatters, or emits, making them the largest category of instrumental methods due to the wide range of radiation types monitored and the significant variation in measurement techniques between methods.

a. **Absorptiometry:** Absorption occurs when a photon hits a molecule, causing it to become excited and decrease in intensity as it travels through the sample. Absorbance spectrophotometry and absorptiometry are used to detect absorption in an assay, as they measure the amount of energy delivered over a unit area in a unit of time.

   Absorptiometry categorizes radiation based on its energy or wavelength range.

   Different types include:

   i. Thermal analysis

ii. Infrared spectrophotometry
iii. Ultraviolet-visible spectrophotometry
iv. X-ray absorption
v. Microwave absorptiometry
vi. Radiowave absorptiometry
vii. Mass spectrometry

These methods measure radiation using different equipment depending on the spectral area, but their working principles remain the same. The radiation is measured using various techniques depending on the spectral area.

Instruments consist of three main components: an electromagnetic radiation source, a transparent cell for holding the sample, and a detector that accurately measures the intensity of the radiation after passing through the sample and cell.

i. **Thermal analysis:** Thermal analysis involves heating an analyte to measure its properties. The sample's temperature is checked during heating, comparing it to an inert material. This data helps identify breakdown processes and is used for qualitative and quantitative analysis.

Thermo gravimetric analysis: TGA records the sample's weight variation in relation to temperature, used in corrosion investigations, alloy and mixture composition analysis, and thermal stability testing.

Differential thermal analysis (DTA): When a sample material is exposed to a controlled temperature program, the temperature difference between it and the material used as a reference is measured as an indication of temperature. Phase diagram development, solid sample phase transition analysis, thermal stability, and polymer characterization.

Differential scanning calorimetry (DSC): When exposed to a certain temperature, the difference in energy inputs between a sample substance and a reference material is measured. used in drug purity analysis and reaction kinetics.

ii. **Infrared spectrophotometry:** Infrared radiation absorption causes vibrational and rotational changes in molecules, reflecting the vibrational energy levels of individual atoms or groups. This technique is commonly used for organic qualitative analysis, as vibrational energy levels depend on atom types and functional groups. However, it can also be used for quantitative analysis by tracking the amount of radiation absorbed at a specific energy peaks in the molecule's spectrum.

iii. **UV-Visible spectrophotometry:** UV-vis spectroscopy (UV-vis) is a widely used method to identify complexes between inhibitory chemicals and electrolyte metals. It provides information on adsorption bands and transitions based on functional groups. Chromophores, molecules that absorb visible or ultraviolet light wavelengths, are present in many compounds. The Beer Lambert law allows for the determination of sample concentration from UV and UV-VIS spectra. UV and UV-VIS spectra are recorded for samples with high and low pH values, and findings are compared to established standards.

iv. **X-ray absorption:** X-ray absorption spectra reveal the energy required to excite electrons from inner orbitals, which are close to the nucleus, to vacant outer orbitals. This energy can ionize an analyte, removing every electron from the atom or molecule. The analysis of X-ray absorption spectra provides information about specific atoms within a molecule, rather than the molecule as a whole.

X-ray absorption is used for qualitative and quantitative analysis, comparing an analyte's spectrum to recognized compounds. The methodology remains consistent across all spectrum areas, with the same measuring procedures used for both qualitative and quantitative analysis.

v. **Microwave absorptiometry:** Electron resonance is studied using spectrometry, which absorbs microwave radiation and changes electron spin states. This method is useful for studying the compositions and behaviors of materials with unpaired electrons. The absorbed radiation can also alter the rotational energy levels of molecules, representing the various ways a molecule can rotate around its chemical link. The allowed rotational levels depend on the types of linked atoms, making it a valuable tool in molecule research.

vi. **Radiowave absorptiometry:**

NMR: Atoms' spinning nuclei can change spin states when exposed to enough energy in a radiofrequency region with a magnetic field. Nuclear magnetic resonance spectrometry can study atomic nuclei and potential spin states, as different atoms have distinct potential spin states with different energy separations. Detecting spin states requires an external magnetic field, as it is only possible when an external magnetic field is present.

The intensity of a magnetic field influences the energy at which absorption occurs, which can be influenced by factors such as neighboring atoms' spinning nuclei. This can shift absorption energies slightly, allowing for the inference of distinct nuclei groups bonded to the atom. Nuclear magnetic resonance spectrometry is particularly useful for qualitative analysis of organic substances, as it helps to determine the quantity and types of these distinct nuclei.

vii. **Mass spectrometry:** Mass spectrometers convert molecules into ions, controlled by magnetic and electric fields. Three key elements are needed: an ion source, a mass analyzer, and a detector. The ion source ionizes the sample, the mass analyzer sorts ions based on their mass-to-charge ratio (m/z), and the detector displays the detected ions on a mass spectrum chart. Most results are expressed in terms of m/z, where z represents the number of charges and m is the ion's molecular weight.

Mass spectrometry (MS) is a powerful analytical method for identifying and measuring therapeutically significant analytes, particularly proteins or peptides with multiple ionic charges. It allows for qualitative and quantitative measurement of a wide range of analytes, extending its capabilities to various clinical applications when combined with gas or liquid chromatographs.

b. **Scattered radiation:** The second primary spectrum technique uses radiation to examine an analyte's particles, scattering them in various directions. The intensity of the incoming or dispersed radiation is measured by a detector. This technique can be used for qualitative or quantitative analysis, depending on the scattering mechanism. If the intensity is determined, a working curve representing the intensity is created for quantitative analysis.

i. **Turbidometry and Nephelometry:** Two methods for quantitative analysis using scattered radiation include turbidimetric measures and absorption measurements. The detector reacts to the lowered intensity of incident radiation if the apparatus is built parallel to the cell and radiative source. Turbidimetric measures measure decreasing intensity, matching findings with absorption measurements. The decreasing intensity is correlated with the concentration of scattering species in the cell at a fixed wavelength, similar to absorption measurements.

Rayleigh and Tyndall scattering methods do not provide qualitative analysis data due to the wavelength of scattered radiation being the same as the incoming light's wavelength. Nephelometry, a technique that measures the intensity of scattered radiation, differs from turbidimetric measurements by positioning the detector perpendicular to the incoming radiation's path, rather than aligned with the radiation source and cell. This makes it impossible to measure the intensity of incident radiation if the detector is in the radiation's path. Tyndall scattering is used in conjunction with nephelometry and turbidimetry to quantitatively assess turbid solutions.

ii. **Refractometry:** Refractometry is a spectral analysis method where the direction of incident light changes. It calculates a substance's refractive index, which is the ratio of electromagnetic radiation's velocity in a vacuum to its velocity in the medium of interest. Measuring velocities of electromagnetic radiation is challenging, so the refractive index is calculated based on the direction of radiation change due to velocity drop. The refractive index, a consistent and precise measure of a material's refraction, is utilized for qualitative examination of pure substances and quantitative examination of simple mixtures with known components.

c. **Emission radiation:** Spectroanalytical techniques use radiation emission measurements after an analyte is initially excited by an external energy source.

i. **Luminescence:** It is the most common scenario, where excitation occurs following electromagnetic radiation absorption. The absorption mechanism is similar to absorptiometric measurements, with an electron in the analyte molecule or atom dwelling in a higher electron orbital with one or more unoccupied orbitals closer to the nucleus. When the excited electron returns to a lower electron orbital, emission occurs, releasing luminescence radiation.

Luminescence occurs when an excited electron returns to the lower electron orbital without flipping its spin or altering its rotation direction when subjected to a magnetic field.

This emission can occur in two ways: after initial absorption, where fluorescence occurs immediately after absorption, and stops as soon as absorption does. However, there is a rare possibility of an excited electron inverting its spin and returning to a lower electron orbital, which is rare.

Phosphorescence refers to the emission of a substance after absorption, which may take time for the spinning electron to flip at the last transition. Both phosphorescence and fluorescence can be used for analysis, but the difference is the duration of the emission delay in fluorescence. Fluorescence ends immediately when stimulating radiation is switched off, while phosphorescence persists.

Phosphorescence is detected in polyatomic species due to electron orbital configurations, while fluorescence is visible in both atoms and polyatomic species. Atomic fluorescence is seen in separate, gaseous atoms. Measurement equipment for fluorescence and phosphorescence is similar to scattered radiation, with detectors often positioned perpendicular to the radiation course. Fluorometers and

phosphorimeters are used to measure fluorescence and phosphorescence, respectively, with phosphorometers tracking luminescence intensity even when light is not hitting the cell.

Luminescence can be caused by various processes, including electromagnetic radiation absorption, flame exposure, atomic emission spectrometry, chemiluminescence, and electrochemiluminescence. Flame emission spectrometry determines the wavelength and intensity of radiation emitted from a flame, while atomic emission spectrometry uses electrical energy to excite an analyte. Chemiluminescence starts luminescence through a chemical reaction, while electrochemiluminescence generates luminescence through an electrochemical reaction.

ii. **X-ray emission:** X-ray emission spectrometry is an analytical technique used to track X-ray radiation emissions. It involves analyzing the emission of X radiation when an electron enters a vacancy in an inner orbital. This vacancy can be created by particle bombardment, nuclear capture, or X-ray absorption. The intensity of the bombardment can remove the atom's inner orbital electron, creating an empty ion.

   X-rays are utilized in surface analysis techniques like particle-induced X-ray emission (PIXE) and proton microprobes. PIXE involves subjecting a sample to particle acceleration and monitoring fluoresced X-rays. Electron microprobes bombard surfaces in scanning electron microscopes, recording the intensity of transmitted or backscattered electrons instead of X-rays. X-ray spectrometers and electron microscopes are often used in tandem to study surfaces.

iii. **Electron spectroscopy:** A collection of analytical techniques known as electron spectroscopy determine the kinetic energy of electrons that are ejected following an initial bombardment of the analyte with X-rays, UV light, ions, or electrons. The analytical technique is known as either X-ray photoelectron spectroscopy (XPS) or electron spectroscopy for chemical analysis (ESCA) when X rays are utilized for the bombardment. The technique is known as ultraviolet photoelectron spectroscopy (UPS) or photoelectron spectroscopy (PES) if the incident light is UV radiation. Auger electron spectroscopy (AES) is the technique used when the impacting particles are electrons and various released electrons are observed. There are further types of electron spectroscopy that are not as commonly employed.

iv. **Radiochemical methods:** Radiochemical technologies detect spontaneous particle emissions or electromagnetic radiation from unsteady atomic nuclei. Quantitative analysis uses the intensity of the radiation, while qualitative studies use the energy. Alpha particles, electrons, protons, neutrons, positrons, and gamma rays can be beneficial in certain situations, with gamma rays originating from nuclear transformations rather than electron orbital changes.

A radioisotope is an elemental isotope that emits radiation or particles. Radioanalytical approaches can analyze radioisotopes, or a nonradioactive sample can be converted into a radioactive substance for testing. A sample can be diluted using a radioactive isotope of the element being tested, and the strength of the emissions from the additional radioisotope can be assayed using isotopic dilution analysis, if the amount of dilution can be calculated.

II. Electroanalytical :

Electroanalysis is a subset of instrumental analysis that uses electrodes to establish an electrical connection with an analyte solution. These electrodes measure an electrical parameter of the solution in combination with electrical equipment. The quantity or identity of the analyte in the solution is correlated with the measured parameter.

Electroanalytical procedures are categorized into:

a. Potentiometry

b. Amperometry

c. Conductometry

d. Electrogravimetry

e. Voltammetry (and polarography)

f. Coulometry

Potentiometry measures voltage by keeping the electric potential constant between electrodes. Amperometry maintains a steady voltage while tracking current. Conductometry analyzes a solution's conductance while keeping electrodes at a constant AC voltage. Electrogravimetry weighs material on electrodes, while voltammetry measures current and potential periodically. Polarography is a type of voltammetry using a liquid metal electrode. A technique called coulometry keeps track of how many coulombs of electricity are used up while the analyte is involved in an electrochemical process.

Most electroanalytical techniques involve electron passage between an analyte and electrodes, with the analyte either donating or removing electrons.

III. Separative technique:

Separation techniques, such as mass spectrometry and chromatography, are crucial for chemical analysis, with mass spectrometry and chromatography being two of the most important.

a. **Chromatography:** An essential biophysical method for both qualitative and quantitative analysis, chromatography allows the components of a mixture to be separated, identified, and purified.

Chromatography, a quantitative analysis method, aims to achieve acceptable separation in a suitable timeframe through the development of various chromatographic techniques.

Several techniques are available for chromatography such as:

i. Gel permeation chromatography
ii. Column chromatography
iii. Thin-layer chromatography (TLC)
iv. Paper chromatography
v. Gas chromatography
vi. Ion exchange chromatography
vii. High-pressure liquid chromatography
viii. Affinity chromatography
ix. Supercritical fluid chromatography
x. Flash chromatography

i. **Gel permeation chromatography:** The method involves using dextran-containing materials to separate macromolecules based on their molecular sizes. In a gel-permeation column, stationary phase consists of inert molecules with small pores. Solutions containing different dimensions are passed continuously with a constant flow rate through the column. Molecules larger than pores cannot permeate into gel particles and are retained between particles. Larger molecules pass through spaces between porous particles and move rapidly inside the column. Molecules smaller than pores diffuse into pores, leaving the column with longer retention times.

ii. **Column chromatography:** Proteins vary in size, shape, net charge, stationary phase, and binding capability. Chromatographic techniques, such as column chromatography, can purify these elements. This method involves separating samples by placing them in a stationary phase column and applying wash buffer as the mobile phase. The inside column material is supported by fiberglass, and samples are collected at the device's bottom in a volume- and time-dependent manner.

iii. **Thin-layer chromatography (TLC):** Thin-layer chromatography is a method used for solid-liquid adsorption, where a solid adsorbent material is placed on glass plates as the stationary phase. This technique can be used with materials like cellulose, silica gel, and alumina. The mobile phase passes through the stationary phase and ascends through capillary action, pushing the mixture onto the plate. Analyte separation is achieved, and the upward traveling rate depends on the solvent's, solid phase's, and material's polarity.

   The chromatogram can be used to determine the locations of colorless molecules in a sample using florescence, radioactivity, or a specific chemical. Visible color formation can be observed in UV and room light. The positions of molecules in the mixture can be determined by determining the ratio between the molecules' lengths and the solvent. The relative mobility is represented by the sign Rf.

iv. **Paper chromatography:** Paper chromatography uses a saturated layer of cellulose as the support material, forming a stationary "liquid phase" of water droplets in the pores of a thick filter paper. The mobile phase is a suitable fluid in a developing tank, making it a type of "liquid-liquid" chromatography.

v. **Gas chromatography:** Gas chromatography is a method used for the precise separation of small compounds. It involves a stationary phase in a column, holding a liquid stationary phase adsorbed onto an inert solid's surface. The carrier phase is He or N2, and the mobile phase is an inert gas forced through a column at high pressure. The sample is then moved into the gaseous mobile phase, and its constituents are distributed between the stationary and mobile phases. This technology is straightforward, versatile, highly sensitive, and quickly applied.

vi. **Ion exchange chromatography:** Ion-exchange chromatography is a method that uses electrostatic interactions between charged protein groups and a solid support material (matrix). Ionic ties increase protein affinity, and the matrix contains an ion load opposite to the protein to be separated. Proteins are extracted from the column by adjusting pH, ion salt concentration, or ionic strength. Anion-exchange matrices adsorb positively charged proteins, while cation-exchange matrices adsorb positively charged proteins.

vii. **High Performance liquid chromatography:** This chromatographic method enables quick purification and structural and functional characterization of various compounds, including proteins, steroids, lipids, carbohydrates, nucleic acids, and other physiologically active substances. The mobile phase in HPLC flows through columns at a high flow rate of 0.1–5 cm/sec while operating at an ambient pressure of 10–400. This method improves the separation power of HPLC and completes the analysis quickly by using tiny particles and applying high pressure to the rate of solvent flow.

viii. **Affinity chromatography:** This chromatography is used for purifying enzymes, hormones, antibodies, nucleic acids, and certain proteins. The filler material is bound by a ligand that forms a compound with proteins like extract, polyacrylamide, and cellulose. The protein that forms a complex with the ligand is bound to the solid matrix, and the bound protein is released from the column by adjusting pH or adding a salt solution.

ix. **Supercritical fluid chromatography:** Supercritical fluid chromatography (SFC) is a method similar to high performance liquid chromatography (HPLC) that uses a non-polar fluid near or above its critical temperature and/or pressure for most of the mobile phase. This fluid has reduced viscosity and increased solute diffusivity, making it more gas-like than typical liquids. SFC separation times can be as short as one-tenth of HPLC separation times. To elute polar solutes, polar organic solvents are combined with non-polar primary fluids, and the polarity range can be extended by more polar additives. For semi-preparative and preparative chromatography of chiral and other tiny, drug-like compounds, SFC is becoming the method of choice.

x. **Flash chromatography:** Clark Still of Columbia University introduced flash chromatography, commonly referred to as medium-pressure chromatography, several years ago (1978). The concept is to quickly force a liquid eluent—typically nitrogen or compressed air—through a small glass column while it is under gas pressure. An adsorbent with a large inner diameter and specified particle size is put within the glass column. While packing with different particle sizes can be utilized, silica gel (40–63 m) is the most widely employed stationary phase. Mostly employed for the isolation and separation of natural components

References

1. Freddy Adams, Mieke Adriaens, The metamorphosis of analytical chemistry Feature Article, 17 December 2019, volume 412, pages3525–3537.
2. Ranga.nr, What is Analytical Chemistry? How is it Important in Daily Life, March 24, 2021 (studyread.com)
3. Miguel Valcarcel, Principles of Analytical Chemistry, Springer Science & Business Media January 2018, pages1–38
4. Elina Sile, lecture-Introduction in analytical chemistry, Basics of analytical chemistry- Academia.edu
5. Jonas Berguist and Charlotte Turner, Analytical chemistry for a sustainable society-trends and implications, Analytical and Bioanalytical Chemistry, 2018, volume 410, pages 3235-3237.

CHAPTER 2

Introduction to Hyphenated Techniques

Introduction

Hyphenated approaches leverage the benefits of both spectroscopic and chromatographic procedures. Pure or almost pure portions of the chemical components of a mixture are produced via chromatography. Selective information for recognition using standards or reference spectra is produced by spectroscopy.

Hirschfeld used the word "hyphenation" a few decades ago to describe the online fusion of a separation technique with multiple spectroscopic detection techniques. This method, which was created by combining spectroscopic detection and separation techniques, is today referred to as the hyphenated method.

Hyphenated approaches have drawn more and more attention lately as the primary method for resolving challenging analytical issues. Over the years, it has been shown that the combination of spectroscopic methods and separation technologies may be used to analyze unknown chemicals in complicated herbal products extracts or fractions in both quantitative and qualitative ways.

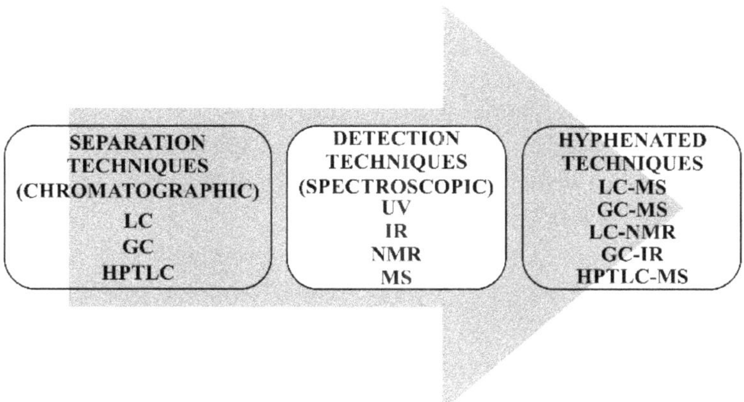

Fig.2.1 Hyphenated techniques.
https://images.app.goo.gl/HZK5cymej7ax1uqJ9

Liquid chromatography (LC), typically high-performance liquid chromatography (HPLC), gas chromatography (GC), or capillary electrophoresis (CE), is used in conjunction with spectroscopic detection techniques, such as Fourier-transform infrared (FTIR), photodiode array (PDA) UV–VIS absorbance or fluorescence emission, mass spectroscopy (MS), and nuclear magnetic resonance spectroscopy (NMR), to obtain structural information that leads to the identification of the compounds present in a crude sample. This allows for the introduction of various modern hyphenated techniques, such as CE-MS, GC-MS, LC-MS, and LC-NMR.

For the qualitative and quantitative identification of chemicals in natural product extracts, high performance liquid chromatography (HPLC) is the most used analytical separation method. The capacity to solve structural issues with complicated natural products has risen due to the physical link between HPLC and NMR or MS. Compared to LC-NMR, LC-MS has been employed more widely because to its higher sensitivity. Hyphenation is not necessarily required to occur between two techniques; many separation or detection techniques, such as LC-PDA-MS, LC-MS-MS, LC-NMR-MS, LCPDA-NMR-MS, and so on, can be coupled together. Large volume injection (LVI), solid-phase microextraction, or on-line coupled with solid-phase extraction (SPE) might be included to provide a more potent integrated system where trace analysis and analyte enrichment are crucial.

The separation and purification of chemicals found in crude extracts or fractions derived from diverse natural sources, as well as the easy recognition of the separated compounds, are the two fundamental components of natural product research. As a result, a high level of sophistication, richness of molecular information, responsiveness, and selectivity are required for the online characterisation of secondary metabolites in pure natural product extracts or fractions. Natural product researchers now have access to incredibly potent new tools that can provide both excellent separation efficiency and the obtaining of on-line identical spectroscopic data on an LC or GC peak that is relevant within a complex mixture, due to the introduction of various hyphenated techniques.

Hyphenated techniques are more appealing and also broadly applicable in nearly all sectors of science, the biological sciences, geographical areas, engineering, agriculture, etc. when chromatographic and spectroscopic techniques are coupled.

Further investigation into the coupling of additional innovative analytical techniques is necessary to enhance the productivity of bioscientific applications and investigations.

List of Double hyphenated techniques:

1. Liquid chromatography-Mass Spectrometry
2. Gas chromatography-Mass Spectrometry
3. Liquid chromatography-Nuclear Magnetic Resonance
4. Gas chromatography- Nuclear Magnetic Resonance
5. Liquid chromatography-Fourier Transform Infrared Radiation
6. Capillary Electrophoresis- Mass Spectrometry
7. Gas chromatography- Fourier Transform Infrared Radiation
8. HPLC-Diode Array Detector
9. Gas chromatography-Atomic Absorption Spectroscopy
10. Inductively Coupled Plasma-Atomic Emission Spectroscopy
11. Inductively Coupled Plasma- Mass Spectroscopy

List of Triple hyphenated techniques:

1. Liquid chromatography -Atomspheric Pressure Ionization- Mass Spectrometry
2. Atomspheric Pressure Chemical Ionization-MS-MS
3. Liquid chromatography - Nuclear Magnetic Resonance-Mass Spectrometry
4. Liquid chromatography – Electron Spray Ionization - Mass Spectrometry
5. Liquid chromatography – Diode Array Detector-Atomspheric Pressure Ionization-Mass Spectrometry
6. Liquid chromatography-Photodiode Array-Mass Spectrometry
7. Liquid chromatography-Photodiode Array- Nuclear Magnetic Resonance- Mass Spectrometry
8. Solid Phase Extraction- Liquid Chromatography-Mass Spectrometry

Advantages:

1. For quick and precise analysis
2. A greater automation levels.
3. Enhanced throughput of samples.
4. Increased repeatability.
5. Because of its closed system, there is lower pollution.
6. Quantification separation concurrently.
7. To resolve challenging analytical issues.
8. Reduced time for study

9. Enhanced combination selectivity, which raises the informational threshold.
10. Offer superior separation efficiency together with online complementary spectroscopy to obtain information on the LC or GC peak of interest in a complicated combination.

References

1. D. Sasipreetam , K. Purna Nagasree , W. Umarani , K. Vara Prasada Rao K and Y. Srinivasa Rao, Review on hyphenated techniques and their applications
2. Kalpesh N Patel, Jayvadan K Patel, Manish P Patel, Ganesh C Rajput, and Hitesh A Patel, Introduction to hyphenated techniques and their applications in pharmacy, Pharm Methods, 2010 Oct-Dec, 1(1): 2–13.
3. Chinaja Godswill Awuchi , Hannington Twinomuhwezi , Chibueze Gospel Awuchi, Chapter 8 - Hyphenated techniques, Analytical Techniques in Biosciences,2022; Pages 125-145
4. Robert Denton Braun, Chemical Analysis, Britannica OzlemCoskun , Separation techniques: Chromatography, North Clin Istanb. 2016; 3(2): 156–160
5. Eshita Garg, Muhammad Zubair, Mass Spectrometer, National Centre for Bio technology Information, January 21, 2023
6. T.A. Berger Chromatography: Supercritical fluid, Theory of Supercritical Fluid Chromatography, Encyclopedia of Separation Science,2007, Pages 1-9

CHAPTER 3

Liquid Chromatography-Mass Spectrometry (LC/MS)

Introduction

The chemical analysis method known as liquid chromatography-mass spectrometry (LC-MS) blends the mass analysis powers of MS with the physical separation capabilities of HPLC. Because of its synergistic qualities, it is widely used in chemical analysis. Because LC-MS has broad coverage of an extensive variety of compounds, it is a viable choice for metabolomics. It can be used in many different fields, such as biotechnology, food manufacturing, medicine, agrochemicals, and the skincare industry. It can also be used in environmental monitoring. Clinical applications using LC-MS have started to be employed since the early 2000s.

An interface in an LC-MS system is used to move divided parts out of the LC columns into the MS ion source. The LC and MS technologies are essentially incompatible, necessitating this interaction. The interface extracts a maximum amount of analyte, transfers the maximum quantity of analyte, and eliminates a sizable amount of the stationary phase utilized in LC. The most widely used LC-MS connections are based on air pressure ionization (API) techniques, which were developed over two decades and were available in the 1990s.

Principle: Mass spectrometry (MS) and liquid chromatography (LC) are two analytical techniques that are combined to form the hyphenated term "liquid chromatography-MS." Using an HPLC, the LC-MS technique separates each component of a mixture separately before ionizing and separating the ions according to their mass/charge ratio. After being separated, the ions are sent to a photo or electron multiplier tube detector, where each ion is identified and measured. The ion source is an essential component of any MS analysis since it effectively facilitates the efficient production of ions for analysis. Ion sources for ionizing intact molecules include ESI (Electron spray Ionization), APCI (Atmospheric Pressure Chemical Ionization), and others. The choice of ion source also depends on whether the target analyte is polar or non-polar chemically.

Instrumentation of LC-MS:

Components of LC-MS

1. Reservoir
2. Pump and gradient controller
3. Injector
4. Pre-column
5. Analytical column
6. Detector
7. Interfaces
8. Mass analyzers

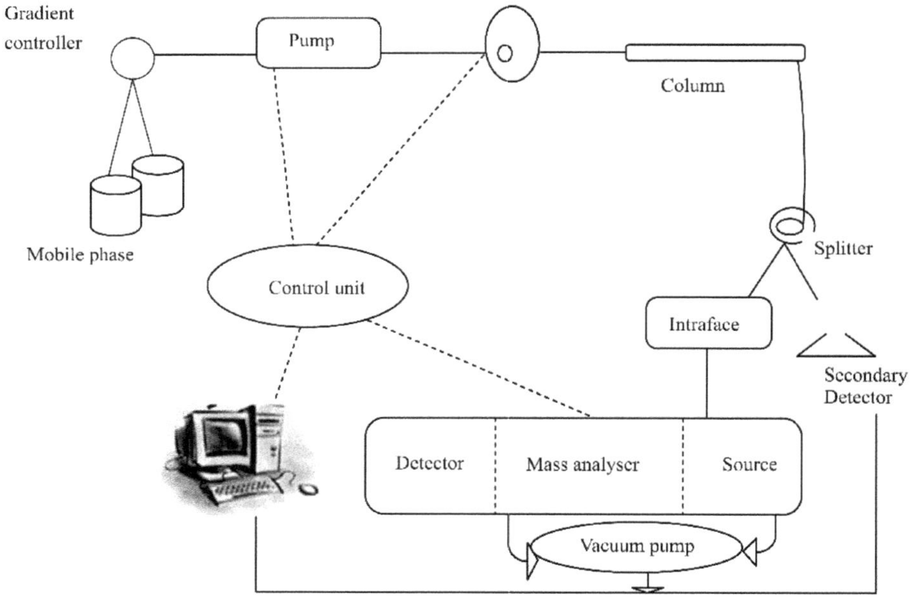

Fig.3.1 Instrumentation of LC-MS.

https://www.researchgate.net/figure/Instrumentation-of-LC-MS_fig2_282121751

1. **Reservoir**: Inert to different aqueous and non-aqueous mobile phases; • Glass or stainless-steel containers that may carry up to 1 Liter of mobile phase (pure solvents made from organic matter or water-based solutions of salts and buffers). The mobile phase undergoes filtration to remove particulate particles and is further degassed by helium sparging, sonication, and vacuum. When using solvents that include halide ions, stainless steel should be avoided.

2. **Pumps gradient controller:** They deliver mobile phase with high pressure. They contain inert solvents. Three major types of pumps are used.

1. **Reciprocating pump:** Inverse flow rates of 1–15 cm^3 per minute can be produced by a reciprocating pump against column backpressures of up to 7250 psi. The pump head, which includes a piston and a solvent chamber with two check valves and a capacity as small as 0.01 cm^3, is the heart of the device. Valve one opens as the main piston exits the chamber, allow the mobile phase to enter the pump head, while valve two closes, stopping liquid from flowing out of the column. Valves one and two close as the piston makes its return stroke into the chamber and open as mobile phase is injected into the column. This procedure is repeated frequently enough to create the desired flow throughout the column.

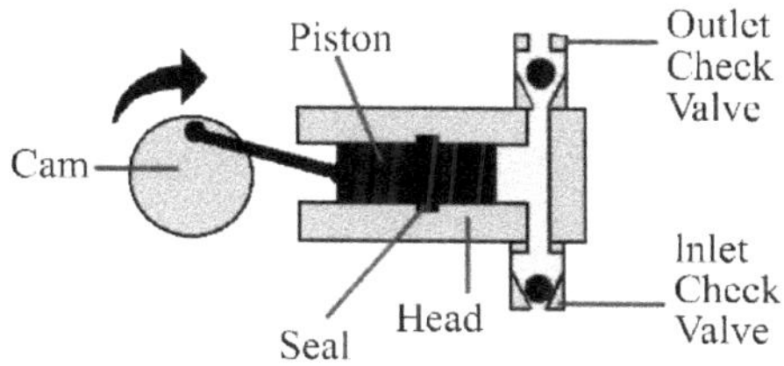

Fig.3.2 Reciprocating pump.
https://www.instructables.com/Simple-reciprocating-pump/

2. **Syringe pump:** These pipes work on the idea of a piston being mechanically moved at a steady pace to displace the solvent in a chamber with a 500 cm^3 volume. These pumps produce a pulse-free flow at high pressures (200–475atm).

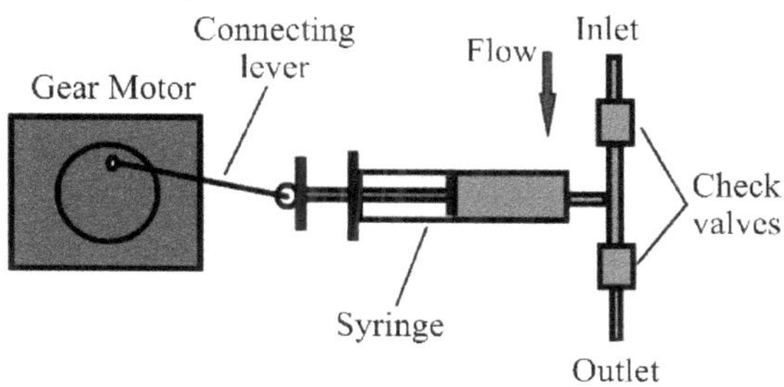

Fig.3.3 Syringe pump.
https://images.app.goo.gl/1FJRq7TWH5mJL8Xq6

3. **Constant pressure pumps:** Also called as gas displacement pump. These pumps offer non pulsating flow. These pumps have low solvent capacity.

   Gradient controller: A pure solvent or a combination of solvents is used to prepare the mobile phase in an isocratic separation. i.e., the same polarity or eluting power of solvent is employed. However, the solvent's polarity is gradually raised in the gradient elution approach, necessitating a change in the solvent's composition. Therefore, when two or more solvent pumps are employed for such separations, a gradient controller is needed.

3. **Injectors:** The chromatographic system's sample volume is introduced using an injector. Typically, a sample volume between 1 and 100 Liters can be injected. The injector loop allows for an increase in injection volume of up to 2 ml. There are a number of injector devices that can be used to manually or automatically inject the sample, including:
   - **(a) Septum injectors:** Also called syringe injection, which are used to inject the sample through a rubber septum or self -sealing elastomer septum. Since the septum must resist high pressures, this type of injector cannot be used frequently.
   - **(b) Stop flow injector:** In this design, the sample is injected through a valve after the mobile phase flow has been temporarily stopped.

4. **Precolumn:** The precolumn is coated with a high percentage of stationary phase liquid to saturate the mobile phase in order to prevent the stripping of stationary phase coated on solid material by the mobile phase. Trap particulate matter in mobile phase and this extends the life of main analytical column; this is why it is called Guard column or Precolumn Filter. Stationary phase is permanently bonded to the support material in banded phase chromatography, so there is no chance of stripping. This is similarly packed with stationary phase to the main analytical column, but the particles are larger.

5. **Analytical column: (Heart of the LC):** The choice of column determines whether analysis is successful or unsuccessful. It was constructed from stainless steel tubes with a diameter of 2-4.6 mm and a length of 5 to 25 cm. The column is filled with 5–10 micron-sized particles. Silica gel is employed as a solid support in analytical columns. Alumina, Diatomaceous earth and activated charcoal are additional materials that may also be used. Sodium silicate is acidified to create silica gel, which is then washed with water. Silica gel's surface contains silanol groups. When the mobile phase is driven through the column, certain components adhere to or diffuse into the packing particles, causing the separation.

6. **Detector:**
   - UV-Visible detector
   - Refractive index detector
   - Fluorescence detector
   - Electrochemical and Conductivity detector
7. **Interfaces:** A combination of liquid components, often including acetonitrile, methanol, and water, are separated using liquid chromatography. The mass spectrometer's ion source receives this liquid that contains a complex variety of components. The ion source is at a high vacuum, therefore different types of interfaces are used.

Moving-belt Interface: The LC column output was deposited in a band on this interface, which was made up of a never-ending moving belt. By properly exhausting the solvent vapours at low pressure in two vacuum chambers while gently heating the solvent, the solvent was efficiently evaporated on the belt. The analytes were flash desorbed into the MS ion source after the liquid phase was eliminated by passing the belt through a heater. The magnetic sector and quadrupole instruments were the MS systems that were most frequently used to link to LC columns via MB interface. MS has been widely used in the investigation of pharmaceuticals, pesticides, steroids, alkaloids, and polycyclic aromatic hydrocarbons because of the MBI interfaces for LC-MS. This interface is no longer in use because to its mechanical complexity, challenges with belt replacement, incapability to handle highly labile proteins, and other factors.

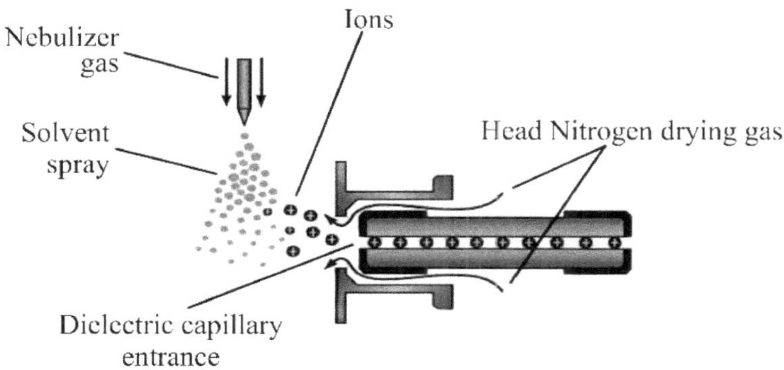

Fig.3.4 Electron Spray Ionization (ESI).
www.researchgate.net/figure/Schematic-diagram-showing-how-electrospray-ionization-works-B1_fig3_266233961

The liquid chromatography (LC) eluent flows through a metal capillary that is located inside the probe during electrospray ionization (ESI). As the

LC flow exits the electrospray capillary, it nebulizes into a spray, which then condenses into droplets. By creating a significant (2–5 kV) potential difference among the electrospray capillary and counter electrode, a charge is imparted onto the droplets. By using a hot drying gas to evaporate the mobile phase, the droplet size is reduced. The charge on the surface density of the smaller droplets is increased by this desolvation. Droplet fission is caused by electric repulsion brought on by the charge density. Coulombic fission occurs when this value far exceeds the droplet's surface tension. Gas-phase ions are created as the droplet "explodes" and are normally sampled through some type of opening. Coulombic fission occurs when this exceeds the droplet's tension at the surface. The generation of protonated or deprotonated molecules with minimum fragmentation, which is optimal for the selection of precursor ions and for maximizing sensitivity, is the main benefit of using ESI for quantitative LC-MS.

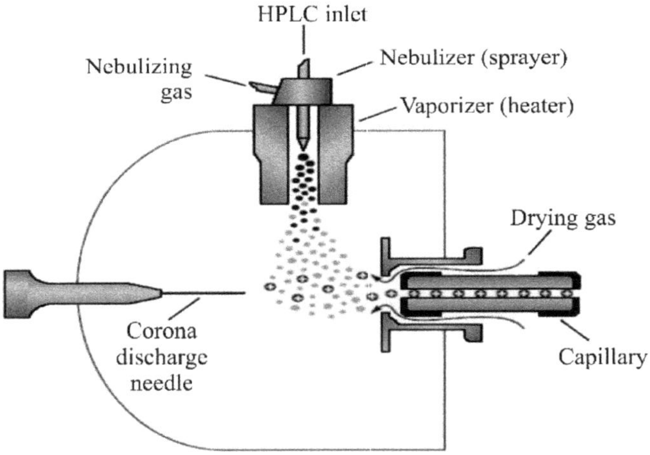

Fig.3.5 Atmospheric Pressure Chemical Ionization (APCI).
analyticalsciencejournals.onlinelibrary.wiley.com/doi/abs/10.1002/mas.10060

APCI stands for atmospheric pressure chemical ionization. In APCI, the LC eluent is sprayed at atmospheric pressure over a heated (usually 250°C–400°C) vaporizer. The liquid is vaporized by the heat. Electrons released from a corona needle ionize and produce gas-phase solvent molecules. Chemical ionization is the process by which the solvent ions impart charge to the analyte molecules. A capillary sample opening allows the analyte ions to enter the mass analyser.

A large variety of polar and nonpolar compounds can be used with APCI. Usually employed for molecules less than 1,500 u, it rarely leads to repeated charging. This makes APCI less suitable than electrospray for the investigation of large macromolecules that can be thermally unstable, in addition to the fact that it involves elevated temperatures.

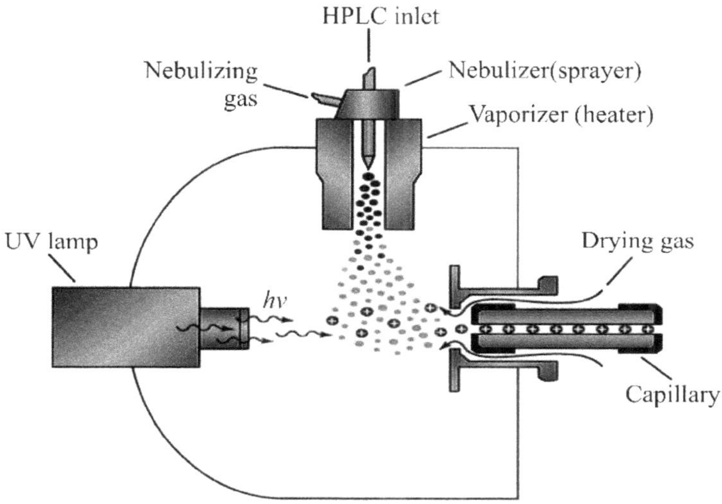

Fig.3.6 Atmospheric Pressure Photo Ionization (APPI).
www.sciencedirect.com/science/article/abs/pii/S0003267008010507

A relatively new method is atmospheric pressure photoionization (APPI) for LC/MS. A vaporizer transforms the LC eluent to the gas phase similarly to APCI. The Photons are produced by a discharge lamp within a constrained range of ionization energies. In order to ionize as many analyte molecules as feasible while reducing the ionization of solvent molecules, the range of energies was carefully selected. The resultant ions enter the mass analyser through a capillary sampling aperture.

8. Mass analyzers:

1. Quadrupole
2. Ion trap mass analyzer
3. Time of flight
4. Fourier transform ion cyclotron resonance.

1. **Quadrupole:** The quadrupole mass filter is the mass analyzer that is used the most frequently. Four solid rods with circular or hyperbolic cross sections that are evenly spaced apart and perpendicular to the ion route make up the quadrupole. Instead of using magnetic fields like the magnet-sector mass spectrometer does, the quadrupole uses electric fields to differentiate the ions according to their m/z. By applying a combination of radio frequency (RF) and direct-current (DC) voltages with the opposite polarity to each rod on the pairs of opposite rods, isolation is achieved. By adjusting the field strengths, it is possible to separate ions with stable oscillations from those with unstable oscillations, causing the former to strike a rod, become neutral, and then be drawn out of the analyzer by the vacuum system.

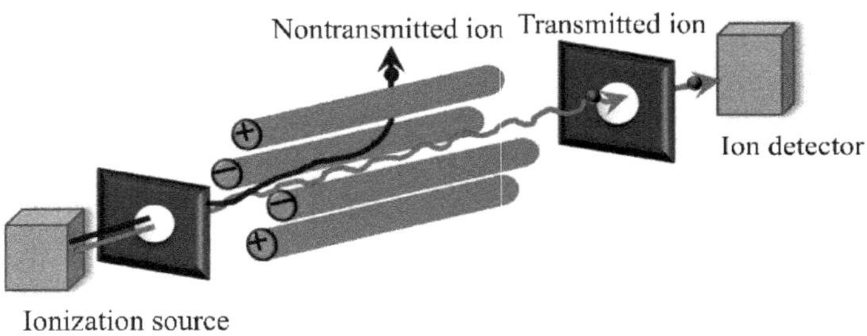

Fig.3.7 Quadrapole.

https://images.app.goo.gl/PQfLFviKz2HUebbk9

2. **Ion Trap Mass Analyzer:** A circular ring electrode and two endcaps that together form a chamber make up an ion trap mass analyzer. Electromagnetic fields inside the chamber act as a "trap" for ions entering the space. To choose which ions are ejected from the trap, use a different field. With ion traps, numerous phases of the mass spectrometry procedure can be carried out without the need for additional mass analyzers.

3. **Time of Flight:** In a time-of-flight (TOF) mass analyzer, all ions are simultaneously subjected to a uniform electromagnetic force, which accelerates them down a flight tube. The mass-to-charge ratios of the ions are calculated by their entry times since lighter ions travel more quickly and arrive at the detector first. Time-of-flight mass analyzers are capable of measuring a wide variety of masses with high precision.

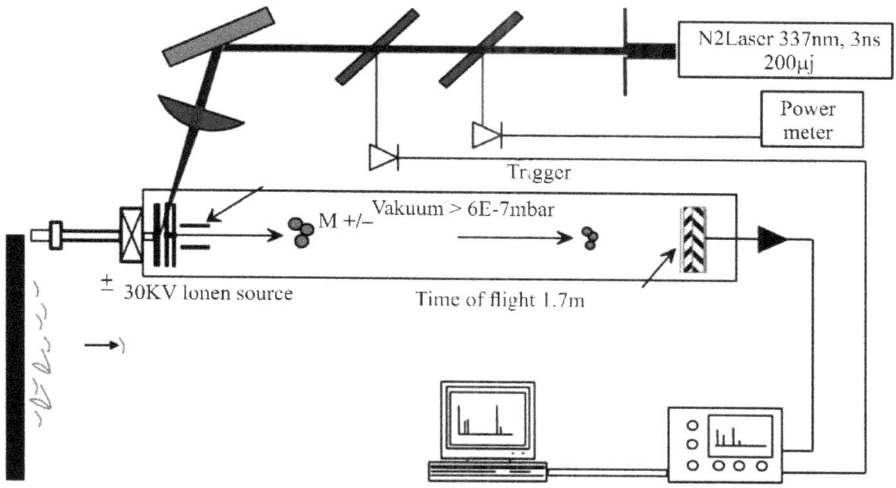

Fig.3.8 Time of flight.
https://images.app.goo.gl/MgFB6dYzaGKLhNFV7

Advantages:

- The most reliable analytical method, LC-MS gives increased sensitivity and selectivity needed to detect an exact molecular weight of a variety of materials. This is its main advantage.
- This can aid pharmaceutical manufacturers in streamlining their research and analysis procedures and ensuring regulatory compliance.
- The two analytical methods (MS and HPLC) are combined to decrease experimental error and increase accuracy.
- In the pharmaceutical, biopharmaceutical, research, forensic, food, and environmental sectors, LC-MS is frequently used to ensure regulatory compliance.
- In comparison to other chromatography methods, the LC-MS provides great selectivity, resolution, exact mass, and specificity.

Disadvantages:

- The main drawback of LC-MS is that it can only be used with volatile buffers, which are necessary for avoiding the API interface from becoming clogged.
- Another drawback of LC-MS is that ionization of the residual contaminants is required before analysis.

- The most used solution in the development of HPLC methods is phosphate buffer, yet phosphate buffer is incompatible with LC-MS analysis.
- In terms of initial expenditures as well as analysis costs, LC-MS is an expensive procedure.
- This is not a mobile instrument; it needs more space and specific handling.
- A qualified individual is needed to operate and analyze data from liquid chromatography and mass spectrometry (LC-MS).

In comparison to other instruments for analysis, the LC-MS requires a lot of care.

Applications:

- Applications for LC/MS range from environmental analysis to the development of pharmaceuticals. It has gained popularity in a number of disciplines due to its exceptional sensitivity and specificity in the detection of a broad spectrum of chemicals.
- Molecular Weight Determination: Determining molecular weights is one of the most basic uses of LC/MS.
- As liquid chromatography may separate delicate and complicated natural mixtures, whose chemical composition needs to be clearly defined (e.g., biological fluids, environmental materials, and pharmaceuticals), a combination of MS with LC systems is appealing. Additionally, the analysis of volatile explosive residues can be done using LC-MS. More than 85% of natural chemical compounds are polar and thermally labile, making LC-MS one of the most used chemical analysis methods today because GC-MS cannot analyze these samples.
- Biochemical Screening for Genetic Disorders
- Used in Therapeutic Drug Monitoring and Toxicology
- Used in identification of bile and metabolite

References

1. De Hoffmann, Edmond Stroobant, Vincent, Mass Spectrometry (Principles and Applications) 2nd edition, 2002, pages 157–158.
2. Pitt, James J, Principles and Applications of Liquid Chromatography–Mass Spectrometry in Clinical Biochemistry, Clin Biochem (February 2009), pages 19–34.

3. Zhou, Bin; Xiao, Jun Feng, Leepika Resscm, Habtom W, LC–MS–based metabolomics, Molecular BioSystems, Feb 2012, Pages 470–481.

4. Chaimbault, Patrick, The Modern Art of Identification of Natural Substances in Whole Plants, Springer, 2014-01-01, Pages 31–94.

5. Dass, Chhabil, Hyphenated Separation Techniques, Fundamentals of Contemporary Mass Spectrometry, John Wiley & Sons, 2007-01-01, pages 151–194.

6. Subramani Parasuraman, Anish Rao, An Overview of Liquid Chromatography-Mass Spectroscopy Instrumentation, Pharmaceutical Methods, Vol 5, Issue 2, December 2014.

7. Ho CS, Lam CWK, Chan MHM, Cheung, Electrospray ionisation mass spectrometry: principles and clinical applications, Clin Biochem, 2003, pages 24:3–12.

Questions

1. What is the principle involved in LC-MS and write advantages disadvantages of LC-MS?
2. Write a note on mass analyzers and interfaces of LC-MS.
3. Add a note on TOF and Quadrupole with neat labelled diagram.

CHAPTER 4

Liquid Chromatography-Nuclear Magnetic Resonance Spectroscopy (LC-NMRS)

Introduction

When combined with detectors such as UV absorption, fluorescence, and electrochemical detectors, high performance liquid chromatography (HPLC) is an effective technique for isolating complex mixtures and can reveal structural information about certain compounds. NMR is an effective technique for learning the intricate structures of organic materials, but because of component interference, analysis results can be challenging to interpret. The mid-to-late 1990s saw the development of HPLC-NMR technology, a sophisticated analytical technique for mixture structural identification, particularly of unknowns. Hyphenated techniques are gaining popularity as high-throughput analytical methods for separating mixtures and obtaining detailed structural information. They combine spectrometric and chromatographic techniques online. However, compared to LC-MS, they are not as widely used and their practicality and operability in manufacturing and research have not been sufficient.

However, there have been significant positive developments since the 2000s, and as a result, LC-NMR is now a very useful analytical technique. This is due to the sensitivity of NMR devices, such as heavily magnetic field magnetic objects and highly sensitive sensors, as well as the maturation of peripheral innovations, like The solvent the reduction technology and naturally measuring software that is appropriate for multi-component analysis. For instance, application for pharmaceutical, chemical, and agricultural research and development. In recent years, additional combination technologies have emerged that allow LC-NMR to be linked with other detectors, making it possible for collecting multiple spectra at once.

Mixture analysis has long made use of LC and NMR, with their physical coupling being proposed more than 30 years ago. In the late 1970s, Watanabe and Niki conducted the first online LC-NMR experiments, demonstrating stopped-flow measurements of combinations of known compounds. Using normal phase columns, deuterated chloroform, and freon, a military jet fuel was the first real examples of to be examined by LC-NMR. In many different fields, LC-NMR along with LC-MS are useful methods for determining the structure of unknown compounds. These methods are crucial for analyzing products made from natural sources because they often contain difficult-to-separate substances that are closely related. New and creative methods are required to characterize the characteristics of every part of intricate mixtures in a quick and easy process. These days, LC-NMR systems are accessible, and based on the sample's condition during the investigation, various modes of data getting can be used.

Principle: High performance liquid chromatography (HPLC) is a faster method of column liquid chromatography that uses high pressure to force solvents through columns. It separates samples into constituent parts based on the difference in relative affinities between molecules. Nuclear Magnetic Resonance (NMR) is a method that uses an external magnetic field to transfer energy between nuclei at radio frequencies. LC-NMR systems typically consist of an auto sampler, pump, column, and non-NMR detector. Reversed phase columns and binary or tertiary solvent mixtures are used in LC-NMR operations. However, proton in the solvent can hinder the obtaining of an adequate NMR spectrum. The LC-NMR system consists of a conventional HPLC system, coupling interface, and NMR system with a flow probe. The liquid chromatograph separates components in the sample, while the interface injects components into the NMR instrument. The sample is then injected into the high-performance liquid chromatography system, separated, and passed through a conventional detector.

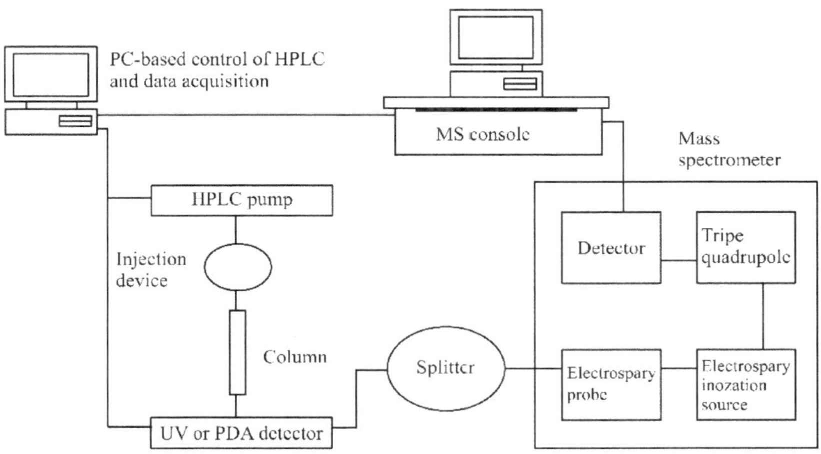

Fig.4.1 Instrumentation of LC-NMR.

https://images.app.goo.gl/fSmThtcMDtnvWyrb7

Components of LC-NMR:

- LC unit
- LC-NMR interfaces
- NMR unit

LC unit: It consists of following parts:

Solvent: According to the makeup of the sample, a glass containing the mobile phase (SAMPLE) will typically contain a combination of polar and non-polar liquid components, each with a different concentration.

Pump: Using a pump, the sample is aspirated out of the the solvent storage facility and pushed through the systems detector and column. A number of variables, such as the stationary phase's particle size, flow rate, and composition, can affect the generation of an operating pressure as high as 42000 kPa, or roughly 6000 psi.

Sample injector: There are two types of injectors: automated and single. An HPLC injector allows for the high-pressure injection of liquid samples under 4000 psi in the volume range of 0.1-100 ml with excellent repeatability.

Column: Particles ranging in size from 3 to 10 um are typically filled with a phase that is stationary. Microbore columns are commonly defined as polished stainless-steel columns with a diameter of less than 2 mm. The mobile phase's temperature and the column unchanged should ideally be maintained throughout the analysis.

Detector: UV spectroscopy, fluorescence, mass spectrometry, and electrochemical detectors are the most often used types of HPLC detectors. The device that detects the analytes that elute from the column of chromatography is situated at the bottom of the column.

Recorders: These are also known as data collection tools. Recorder: Use an electronic integrator or chat recorder to capture the signals coming from the detector. A chromatograph designed to be simple to read and interpret is created by the computer by integrating the detector's response to each component.

LC-NMR interfaces:

Direct coupling: which includes direct flow of LC effluent in to NMR flow cell and continuous recording of spectra.

- Post-Column Splitter

- Value-Switching interface i.e., BNMI (Bruker NMR-mass spectrometry interface)

Indirect coupling: Intermediate storage loop which transfer outlet of LC to NMR flow cell at specified time interval. This can be done by Solid phase Extraction method

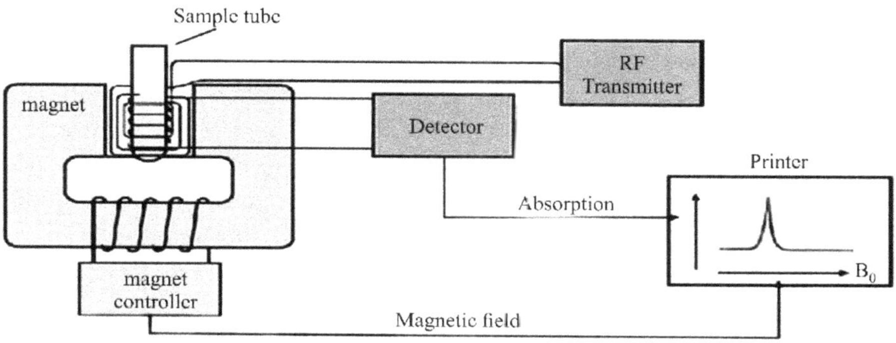

Fig.4.2 NMR unit.

https://images.app.goo.gl/gAVZWVRtguLQLsTa9

It consists of following parts: The following units are involved in NMR instrumentation. To distinguish between the nuclear spin energy state, use a magnet. There are two radio frequency channels: one for providing RF radiation and the other for field/frequency stabilization. A sample probe with coils to connect the sample to the radiofrequency examples of holder, RF oscillator, move generator, and RF receiver make up the field. An observer to handle the signals from NMR. A recorder with a spectrum display.

Magnets: The Magnets are employed to supply the field Ho's principal component, which establishes the Larmor or the frequency at which any nucleus decays. The line increases with increasing magnetic field strength. separation of nuclei with chemical shifts on a frequency scale. The proportionate numbers of the increase in the NMR experiment's sensitivity at lower energy spin levels.

Qualities: It should produce a homogeneous magnetic field, meaning that over extended periods of time, the magnetic field's strength and direction should remain unchanged. At least 20,000 gaus should be the minimum strength of the field.

Varieties of magnets

- Permanent magnets
- Electro magnets and
- Super conducting magnets.

Super Conducting Magnets (SCM): In Nuclear Magnetic Resonance (NMR), superconducting magnets produce a powerful, steady, and uniform magnetic field that is necessary for the precise and accurate detection of nuclear electromagnetic resonant signals. Superconductive materials, including niobium-titanium or niobium-tin, that have been refrigerated to very low temperatures are commonly used in these magnets. This allows the components to carry electrical free resistance and produce intense magnetic fields. At low temperatures (usually less than 6K), the resistance in the superconducting wire becomes zero. The coil is submerged in a bath of superconducting material to keep the wire in that state.

He (Li) in liquid state, While the "heat shield" came into proximity to a bath of inexpensive liquid nitrogen to lessen the quantity of liquid helium that boils off; empty space flask to decreases the heat flow even more.

Magnetic coils: Large stable magnets have a difficult time changing their magnetic fields, but this issue can be solved by overlaying a tiny magnetic field on top of the primary field. A pair of Helmholtz coils, which are instruments for creating an almost uniform.

Magnetic field on the pole encounters of the permanent magnet, named because of the German von Helmholtz carries out this. These coils create a magnetic field that is adjustable by changing the current flowing through them. passing via them. The direction of production of the small electromagnetic field is the same as the and is included in the primary field. Both fields are applied to the sample, and one field appears to the centre.

Probe unit: It is a spectrophotometer system's recognizing component. It is placed between the magnet's pole faces in the X-Y plane of the air gap to adjust the tip of the probe holder. Thus, in a nuclear magnetic resonance experiment, the sample is subjected to the combined effects of two magnetic fields, namely Ho and RF(EMR). Glass is a common material for NMR sample cells because it is affordable and robust. It is made up of a glass tube with a 7.5 cm length and an outer diameter of 5 mm that holds 0.4 ml of liquid. In NMR, the sample tube is held horizontally between the magnet's pole faces. Along with the reference cell, the probe has a sample holder, sweep, and detector coils. The orientation of the detector and receiver coil is 90 degrees apart. The sample tube rotates on its longitudinal axis at a rate of 30 to 40 revolutions per minute thanks to the sample probe. Every component of the specimen tube experiences the field's time average at the same rate.

Radio frequency generator: The radio frequency electromagnetic radiation needed to cause the sample's nuclei to transition from their ground states to their states of excitement is produced using an RF oscillator. The source of noise is a crystal-controlled oscillator that is extremely stable. To achieve the greatest contact with the sample, it is mounted opposite to the magnetic field and at a right angle to the path about the field injuries around the sample tube. The sample is exposed to Rf radiation by the oscillator. Radio frequencies are produced through the technological multiplication of a quartz crystal's inherent frequency, which is housed within a thermally stable block. The oscillator's coil is wound around the sample container to maximize the amount of RF radiation that interacts with the substance being studied.

Shim coils: Line lengths of less than one is necessary for high resolution NMR.A homogeneous magnetic field must be applied across the sample in order to minimize any corresponding variations in the Larmor frequency. To neutralize the slight residual inhomogeneities in the main magnetic field, encircle the specimen with a series of shim coils, every one of which generates a tiny field of magnetic attraction with a distinct geographic profile. Up to 40 distinct shim coils may be found in modern spectrometers. These coils are labeled with the field histories they produce, such as x, y, z, z^2, z^3, xy,xz, yz, x^2-y^2, etc.

Because different shims will interact with one another, optimizing the shims requires skill and experience. This process is called shimming.

The transmitter channel:

Synthesizer: radiofrequency source that generates a precisely adjustable, steady frequency. Using an RF amplifier, increase the power of this weak signal to at least 100W so that it has sufficient energy to stimulate the sample's NMR active nuclei.

Attenuator: The attenuator is a device which lowers a signal's strength level; the power level is usually measured in decibels (dB). An attenuator in a computerized system can be precisely changed and controlled digitally or programmatically to change the intensity of a signal that passes through it.

Modes of LC-NMR:

- **Continuous flow:** Eluent is sampled "real-time" as it passes through the NMR detection coil in a continuous flow (on flow). The NMR probe is immediately attached to the LC-detector's outlet. NMR spectra are constantly obtained as the peaks elute. The samples and peaks are passed across the NMR cell using the chromatographic technique. This operating mode is also achievable with any of the LCNMR interfaces (BPSU / BSFU), They are not necessary, though.
- **Stopped flow:** The pump is stopped where needed, and data is collected. The NMR probe is immediately attached to the LC-detector's outlet. Peaks eluting from the column are detected using an LC-detector, which is typically UV in color. The flow keeps going after a peak is found until it reaches the NMR cell. At this point, the NMR tests are carried out and the chromatography process (pump, gathering data, gradient) is stopped. After the NMR studies are finished, chromatography is carried out again until the following peak is identified. Multiple iterations of this procedure are possible inside a single chromatogram.
- **Time slices:** Interest regions, or "time-slices," are examined.

  It involves halting the flow for brief periods of time during the chromatography peak in order to time slice various portions of the chromatography run. It is helpful when the precise chromatography retention period is unclear, when there is deficient chromatography separation, or when the substance under investigation has a poor or absent UV chromophore. A comprehensive NMR chromatogram (tNMRc) is the resultant data from an experiment where a time slice is conducted.
- **Peak parking:** Off-line sample loops are utilized to "park" points of interest.

  The specimen loops on either BPSU-36 or BPSU-12 are linked to the LC-detector's outlet.

  Peaks dissolving from the column are detected using an LC-detector, usually UV The chromatography is not stopped when an identified peak is moved into one of the sample loops. Upon completion of the chromatography, which the peaks that result from the loops are transferred into the NMR probe using the HPLC pump.

- **Peak trapping:** These samples are "re-concentrated" using Solid Phase The process of ex The SPE unit is linked to the LC-detector's outlet. Peaks eluting off the column are detected using an LC-detector, usually UV in nature. Moving and trapping a detected peak on a SPE cartridge allows for uninterrupted chromatography. Following the completion of the chromatography, the separation solvents are eliminated and the peak is transferred into the NMR probe using completely deuterated solvents. traction cartridges.

Advantages of LC-NMR:

- **Structural clarification:** The blend of separating and structure information that LC-NMR offers is quite effective.
- It enables us to link NMR spectra and chromatographic retention durations directly.
- Together, these efforts aid in the identification and clarification of complicated chemical structures, such as those of metabolites, natural products, and contaminants.
- **Trace component detection:** In complicated mixtures, LC-NMR is highly effective at finding trace components.
- These elements can be recognized and described even in extremely small amounts. This is important for quality control, environmental analysis, and medication development.
- **Insights into metabolomics:** metabolic characteristics are revealed by LC-NMR in metabolomics investigations. Through the examination of eluted chemicals' NMR spectra, scientists can learn more about changes and metabolic pathways.
- It helps in the finding of biomarkers and the understanding of disease mechanisms
- These strategies work extremely differently from one another and do not interfere with other techniques because the information they supply is orthogonal to each other. For example, whereas NMR aids in determining the structure (via various studies), LC procedures aid in the separation of complex mixtures.
- Whether a peak represents a pure or impure substance can be ascertained using NMR.
- NMR data can be obtained even if the mixture is not entirely separated.
- The method is non-destructive.
- The sample can be kept for analysis using a different technique.

Disadvantages of LC-NMR:

- This method entails significant expenses.
- High equipment expenditures are also included in capital.
- More time is needed to complete experimental tasks.
- It additionally involves the partial usage of deterritorialized liquids.
- Operator training requirements stem from the need for qualified workers.
- The challenge of choosing a solvent.

Applications of LC-NMR:

Natural product analysis: Natural product analysis is made easier by LC-NMR technology, which offers tiny amounts, great efficiency, and speed. It gives an overview of complex extracts by describing the relative contents and variations in chemical makeup. With its ability to identify recognized chemicals early and concentrate on structural studies of new compounds, this method is perfect for plant extracts containing various components.

Isomer analysis: In order to identify the structure, concept, and optical isomers, LC-NMR is still crucial. The detection concentration may be accurately determined to nanograms using LC-NMR method for separating and recognizing of stereoisomers that which completely reflects the stereoscopic discriminating capacity of NMR.

Metabolite analysis: Because of the wide dispersion of medications and their metabolites, the small sample sizes, and the non-repeatable nature of the samples, metabolite evaluation is essential to pharmacological research and clinical monitoring. A straightforward, continuous technique that can be used to find possible markers and identify complicated metabolites is LC-NMR.

Polymer analysis: The synthetic polymer is a multi-component, highly complicated material made up of molecules with various chain dimensions, chemical compositions, and structural variations. In addition to separating polymers based on their molecular weight, LC-NMR technology may also differentiate between polymers that have the same molecular mass but distinct branches.

Environmental surveillance: It is possible to precisely identify the kinds and concentrations of different trace chemicals, including ultra-trace compounds, in environmental samples by analyzing them using LC-NMR spectroscopy.

References

1. Subham Kumar Vishwakarma, LC-NMR (Liquid Chromatography-Nuclear Magnetic Resonance), Advanced spectral analysis (MPC201T) August,2021.
2. M. Jaya Sree, Shyamala Mudavath, updated review on LC-NMR, World Journal of Pharmaceutical Research, Volume 8, Issue 2, pages 380-395,27 July 2005

Questions

1. Write a note on instrumentation of LC-NMR.
2. Add a note on applications, advantages and disadvantages of LC-NMR.

CHAPTER 5

Liquid Chromatography-Fourier Transform Infrared Spectroscopy (LC-FTIS)

Introduction

The coupling of liquid chromatography to Fourier transform infrared spectroscopy (LC-FTIR) is a crucial technique for analyzing unknown chemical components in mixtures. Early attempts used offline methods, but the need for faster analysis times, automation, sample throughput, better reproducibility, and lower contamination levels has led to the need for online LC-FTIR instrumentation.

Principle: Liquid chromatography is a technique used in various fields, including food production, judicial proceedings, sports testing, pharmaceuticals, and medical diagnoses, to separate mixtures into distinct components. Infrared spectroscopy, on the other hand, describes functional groups by analyzing the frequencies absorbed by molecules, particularly in distinguishing structural isomers, making it effective in identifying substances.

The easiest method for combining LC with IR spectroscopy is by utilizing a flow cell. While the effluent from the LC column is being cycled through the flow cell, IR spectra are continually being monitored. Real-time detection, low maintenance requirements, and ease of use are just a few advantages of this.

Unfortunately, it is somewhat less desirable due to the usual LC solvents' IR-absorption, which reduces detection sensitivity and the amount of spectral data that can be collected.

Another alternative is to get rid of the LC solvent before using IR detection. In this instance, the effluent is evaporated at an interface before chemicals are deposited on a substrate for IR spectroscopy. It permits more sensitivity but does so at the expense of operating simplicity.

Instrumentation: The main components of LC-FTIR are:

1. Liquid chromatography
2. Interface
3. FT-IR

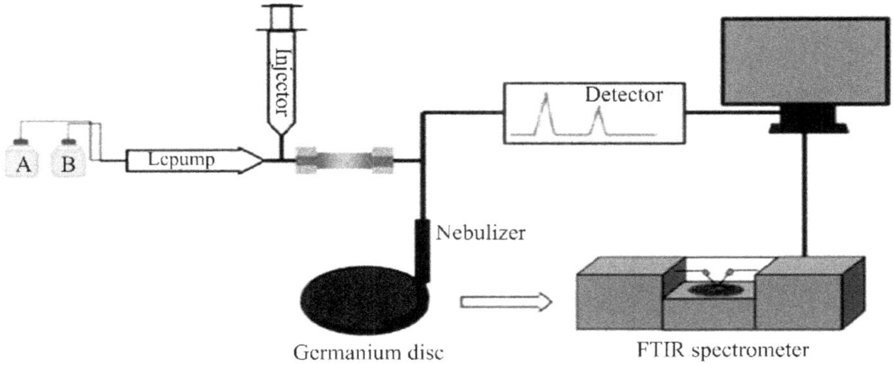

Fig.5.1 Instrumentation of LC-FTIR.
https://images.app.goo.gl/y5NP461cdsHU137TA

1. Liquid chromatography:

A. Reservoir:

It involves the use of glass or stainless steel containers to store up to 1 liter of mobile phase, which is filtered to remove impurities and degassed using vacuum, sonication, and helium sparging, and should not be used with halide ions.

B. Pump and gradient controller:

(a) Mechanical –

1. Reciprocating piston type: Delivers steady flow rate
   Pressure fluctuation may result in an unstable baseline, therefore
2. Use of a pulse damping device

(b) Pneumatic - Produces continuous pressure, operates without pulses, and doesn't need a pulse dampening mechanism.

I. Gas displacement type: This method forces the solvent out of a tube under direct pressure from a highly compressed gas.

II. Amplifier type: Wherein a piston is forced to release liquid by compressed gas at a lower pressure

Gradient controller: A technological tool that coordinates the performance of two pumps to provide a mobile phase mixture with the required concentration.

C. Injector:

- One to one hundred micro liters of fluid can be injected.
- The injector loop allows for an increase in injection volume of up to 2 mL.
- Several injector devices are available for manual or automatic sample injection, including:

(a) Septum injector:

- It is used to inject the sample through the septum, which is made of rubber.
- Since the septum must resist high pressures, this type of injector cannot be used frequently.

(b) Stop flow injector:

In this design, the sample is injected through a valve after the mobile phase flow has been temporarily halted.

(c) Rheodyne injector:

- It has a predetermined capacity of loop for keeping sample until it is introduced into the column, such as 20 µL, 50µL, or more, and is the most extensively used injector.
- The sample is injected into the column by an injector.
- The injector is placed directly before the column's intake.

D. Pre column:

The precolumn, also known as a guard column or precolumn filter, is a column used in banded phase chromatography to trap particles in the mobile phase. It is coated with a high concentration of stationary phase liquid to prevent stripping of solid phase-produced solids.

The column is also used to trap larger particles, which are 2 to 10 cm long, extending the life of the primary analytical column.

E. Analytical column:

- The choice of column is crucial for successful analysis.
- It is made from stainless steel tubes with a diameter of 2-4.6 mm and a length of 5-25 cm.
- The column is filled with 5-10 micron-sized particles and is supported by silica gel, alumina, diatomaceous earth, and activated charcoal.
- The column is acidified to create silica gel, which is then washed with water.
- Separation occurs when components stick to or diffuse into the packing particles, with silanol groups on the surface.

2. Interface:

A. Flow cell interface:

Flow cells simplify the online connection between LC and FTIR by collecting real-time IR spectra by passing the LC's effluent through them. This method offers low cost, simple operation, low maintenance requirements, and the use of non-volatile buffers. Flow-cell detection is useful for online response monitoring as it occurs in real-time, but dynamic IR observations reduce the signal-to-noise ratio (SNR) due to less time for spectra collection.

Types of flow cells:

(a) Transmission cell:

- It is made up of two IR transparent windows or an IR transparent cavity and is spaced apart by a Teflon or metal spacer. Through capillary tubing, the LC eluent enters and leaves the cell, where it is sampled by an IR beam that is traveling perpendicularly.
- When chloroform is utilized as the M.P., the path length is 0.001 to 2 mm, and the detection limits are 40-50 microgram.

(b) Flow cells is based on the ATR principle:

- One kind of cell is made up of an ATR crystal with cone-shaped ends that is cylindrical in shape.
- The cone ends of the crystal are integrated outside the cell body in a flow cell. The effluent travels through the crystal's flow-cell cavity.

(c) Flow cell is based on specular-reflection measurements:

- The device is a stainless-steel cell body with an IR-transparent glass, guiding an IR beam towards the flow-cell window under normal incidence angles. The beam travels through the cell window, is reflected by a mirror, twice traverses the effluent flow channel, and is directed towards the detector by a second external mirror.
- The optical pathlength is twice the thickness of the sample cavity and is directed towards the detector by external second mirror.

B. Solvent elimination interface:

- The process involves removing the eluent, applying it to a nebulizer, depositing the separated analytes on a substrate, and using the immobilized chromatogram to generate IR spectra.
- Compared to flow - cell methods, solvent elimination LC-FTIR methods offer several benefits, including the complete utilization of IR spectroscopy identification potential due to the absence of interfering eluent absorption bands, and the accessibility of the immobilized chromatogram even after the chromatographic run is completed.

Types of Solvent Elimination Interfaces:

Early LC-DRIFT interfaces: The LC eluent was dripped into individual KCl-filled cups using a heated tube, and any remaining solvent was wiped away with a mild nitrogen stream before spectra were acquired.

(a) Buffer memory technique:

For transmission tests, flat KBr plates are employed. On a substrate, an entire chromatogram is immobilized and saved. Eluent was rapidly evaporated using micro-bore LC and low flow rates.

- FTIR transmission microscopy for the acquisition of spectrum.
- Analyte research using X-ray fluorescence spectra.

(b) Spray type interfaces:

I. Thermospray interfaces:

Part of the liquid evaporates to an expanding vapour as it passes through a directly heated vaporized tube, causing a mist of desolvating droplets to emerge at the tube's end.

Temperature functioning between: 100 °C and 300 °C

Limits of detection: 1 mg

II. Particle beam interface:

For the LC-separated substances deposition on the KBr substrate.

Three components:

By nebulizing the LC eluent with He, a monodisperse aerosol is produced. Then it is sent into a desolvation chamber, where the majority of the liquid vapourizes. The interest-specific analyte molecules enter the IR-transparent substrate after being separated. The substrate is then taken out of the vacuum chamber after deposition and brought to the FT-IR spectrometer.

III. Electrospray interface:

A strong electric field is used to generate a spray of charged droplets. Due to solvent evaporation and charge density, the initial droplets further fragment into smaller droplets. ZnSe Plate is the deposit surface.

IV. Pneumonic nebulizer:

This device uses a high-speed gas flow to break up liquid surfaces and create tiny droplets that are then spread by the gas. Surface of Deposit: IR-Reflective Disc, Nitrogen gas, a gas.

V. **Ultrasonic nebulizer:**

By pouring LC effluent onto a transducer that is vibrating at ultrasonic frequencies, a Spray is created. Small, desolvating droplets of the solvent are created by the vibrations and are carried by a carrier gas in the direction of a substrate. KBr discs are the deposition substrate.

3. FT-IR:

A. Interferometer:

The brain of an FTIR spectrometer is the interferometer, which comprises of a beamsplitter, a stationary mirror, and a moving mirror. A semi-transparent mirror called a beamsplitter separates a collimated light beam into two optical channels. Half of the light is reflected onto the stationary mirror, while the other half is transmitted to the moving mirror. The two light beams are reflected by the moving and stationary mirrors, which are then recombined at the beamsplitter before passing through the sample chamber and landing on the detector.

B. Detector:

The transmitted or reflected light from a sample is measured and converted into an electrical signal using FTIR detectors. The kind and composition of the detector influence its sensitivity and the wavelength range of the data it can record.

The beam is transformed by the detector into photons, which are subsequently converted into quantifiable electric signals that the computer can decipher. These are a few illustrations of typical detectors:

- Room temperature DLATGS is a regular analysis tool.
- Sensitive applications use cooled liquid nitroglycerin.
- Visible infrared and near-IR applications use Si-photodiodes.
- Far-infrared bolometers made of silicon

Advantages:

- Elimination of LC solvent before IR detection is used
- Allows enhanced sensitivity
- Cost of ease at operation

Disadvantages:

- Its primary drawback is the solvents frequently employed in LC's substantial IR absorption. Both the detection sensitivity and the available spectrum information are severely constrained by these absorptions.

Applications:

1. Analyzing small amount of sample.
2. Examining environmental toxins such as pesticides, herbicides, and polycyclic aromatic hydrocarbons.
3. Analyses of pharmaceuticals including analgesics and steroids, as well as their impurities, drug metabolites, polymer additives, colors, and fullerenes.
4. Isomer differentiation
5. Dissociation of the secondary structure of proteins like lysozyme and beta globulin.

References

1. Kabita Sharma, Fourier Transform Infrared Spectroscopy (FTIR): Principle, Instrumentation, Applications, Advantages, Limitations, Science info, July 8, 2023
2. A Brief Introduction to LC-IR, Chromatography today, Feb 18 2022
3. Subham Kumar V, Liquid Chromatography- Mass spectrometry, Reasearch gate, August 2021
4. Subham Kumar V, Liquid Chromatography-Fourier-Transform Infrared spectrometry (LC-FTIR), Reasearch gate, August 2021
5. Tania Maria Grazia .S , Carmelo .C, Paola .D , Luigi .M, The online coupling of liquid chromatography to Fourier transform infrared spectroscopy using a solute-deposition interface: A proof of concept
6. Govert Willem. S, Tom .V, Liquid Chromatography/Infrared Spectroscopy, Research gate September 2006

Questions

1. Write a note on interfaces of LC-FTIR.
2. Mention the applications of LC-FTIR.
3. Describe the instrumentation of LC-FTIR.
4. Write drawback of flow cell type interface.

CHAPTER 6

Gas Chromatography-Mass Spectrometer (GC-MS)

Introduction

A gas chromatography is often employed as the analytical instrument, and then it is hyphenated to a mass spectrometer using a heated transfer line. The two operations occur in turn.

Principle: A GC-MS experiment involves sample preparation, injection, and separation on a GC column, with molecules transferred to a mass spectrometer via an interface and ionization chamber for fragmentation of molecules.

A mass analyzer uses a magnetic or electric field to sort ions based on their mass to charge ratio (m/z). It can sort hundreds of distinct ion masses in one second. The detector determines the number of electrons formed when the ions impact the detector, thereby quantifying the ions.

The mass spectrum (MS) is the fundamental MS-specific dimension of data, providing a graphic representation of the abundance of each ion as a function of m/z, serving as a detector for GC.

Instrumentation:

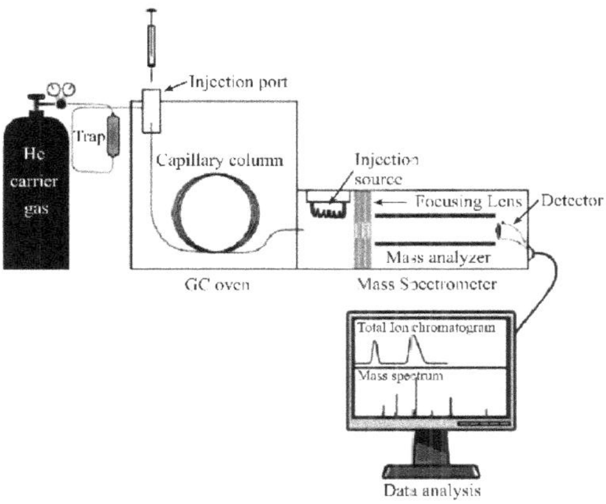

Fig.6.1 Instrumentation of GC-MS.
https://images.app.goo.gl/ApXrs71t6nUgYS9a7

Components of GC-MS:

It mainly consists:

A. Gas Chromatography

1. Carrier gas
2. Injection system
3. Column
4. Oven

B. Mass Spectrometer

1. Ionization
2. Mass Analyzer
3. Vacuum system
4. Detector

A. Gas Chromatography:

1. **Carrier gas:** The carrier gas, or mobile phase, must be chemically inert and is commonly placed in pressurized tanks. The flow rate is regulated by pressure regulators, gauges, and flow meters, with typical flow rates for packed columns being 25-150 mL/min and 1–25 mL/min for open tubular capillary columns.

   The most widely utilized gas is helium, although argon, nitrogen, and hydrogen are also employed.
2. **Injection system:** Samples are inserted as vapor plugs, injected into a heated sample port at 50°C beyond boiling point, and transported to the column using calibrated micro syringes, ensuring proper temperature control.
3. **Column:** Gas chromatography involves sample components traveling through capillary columns coated with stationary phase or silicon particles, typically several meters long (10-120m) or inner diameter (0.10-0.50 mm), compared to packed columns with a diameter of 2-4 mm and length(1-5m).
4. **Oven:** The temperature of the gas chromatographic ovens, which are configurable for temperature, normally ranges from 5℃ to 400℃ but can go as low as -25℃ with cryogenic cooling.

Interfaces: The GC/MS interface is used for attenuating carrier gas, redirecting extra gas into a backup exhaust system, and ensuring the gas chromatographic peak is not broadened.

Most GC/MS interface solutions have an enrichment component, allowing studies in the 1-10 ng range but requiring 90% of the sample, especially for low-level samples.

Membrane separator uses permeability variances to separate gas chromatograph effluent from the mass spectrometer vacuum system. Organic molecules are adsorbed, while helium or other permanent gas has low permeability and is not adsorbed by the membrane.

The membrane's permeability is influenced by solubility and diffusion rate, with helium yield ranging from 30 to 90%. Temperature restrictions and optimization are significant issues, affecting GC/MS work and causing top limits.

The ideal temperature for each substance's solubility and diffusivity tradeoff leads to sample discrimination and a 0.1 second delay, with polar and highly flammable substances often partially adsorbed.

Supersonic jet/orifice systems are efficient in using the effusion principle to remove carrier gas. Gas chromatograph effluent is forced through a tiny opening, expanding and entering a vacuum chamber. The gas stream is guided into a second aligned jet or orifice due to higher helium diffusion rate. Small deviations reduce efficiency.

The separator requires adjustment for different flow rates and can be used in series with two jet/orifice assemblies. It yields around 25% under normal conditions and is ideal for low-capacity mass spectrometers. Single-stage jet/orifice separators are commonly used with packed columns at 30-50 ml/min, with minimal peak distortion.

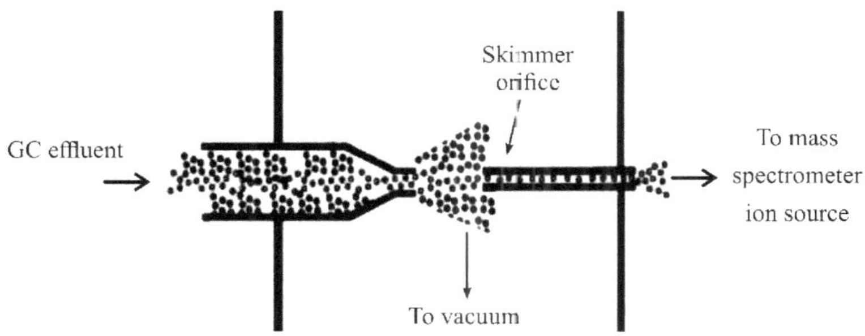

Fig.6.2 Orifice separators
https://images.app.goo.gl/ekwN67kAeuc3pSRK6

B. Mass Spectrometer:

1. Ionization: In this the molecules undergo ionization before being analysed by the detector. Mainly two types of ionizers are used. They are:

Electron Impact (EI): It is a popular method for ionization, where an excess of energy is applied to analyte, causing ion fragmentation. This technique involves creating a high-energy electron beam by applying a voltage to a heated filament. The beam bombards neutral molecules, stripping electrons from their valence shells, and converting some molecules to molecular ions. This results in the formation of radical cations, M+, with the analyte molecule M having a positive charge and the dot representing an unpaired electron.

Electron ionization (EI MS) involves the production of ions from molecular ions, which result in bond cleavage, rearrangement, or fragmentation into mass fragment ions. The vacuum system removes most material and byproducts. EI MS typically uses an electron beam with a potential of 70 eV, necessary for organic compounds under 1000 atomic mass units.

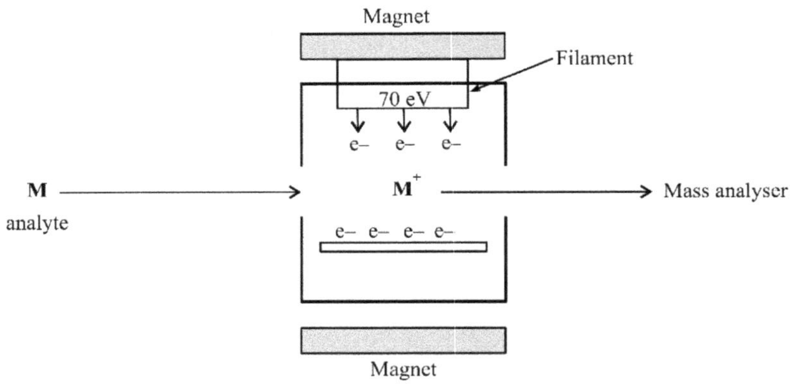

Fig.6.3 Electron Impact.
https://images.app.goo.gl/8qw3YLPjKPdHmH1y7

Electron impact	Electron spray ionization
EI is a hard ionization process, numerous fragments may occur, and occasionally a molecule ion may be lost.	ESI is a soft ionization process. In contrast to there are certain fragments
Low formula mass organic or inorganic compounds are affected by electron impact.	Higher molecular mass compounds, such as biological molecules like proteins, are treated by electrospray ionization.
Samples must be thermally volatile and stable.	Suitable for charged, polar, or basic chemicals

Chemical Ionization (CI): It is a popular soft ionization method Ion-molecule interactions are used in chemical ionization to generate ions from the analyte. When a reagent gas, such methane, isobutane, or ammonia is ionized by electron impact, from there chemical ionization process starts. Ion-molecule reactions between the reagent gas neutrals and ions are caused by a high reagent gas pressure (or lengthy reaction time). Analyte ions can be created when certain byproducts of these ion-molecule interactions react with the analyte molecules. However, EI is the most popular ionization method for GC-MS.

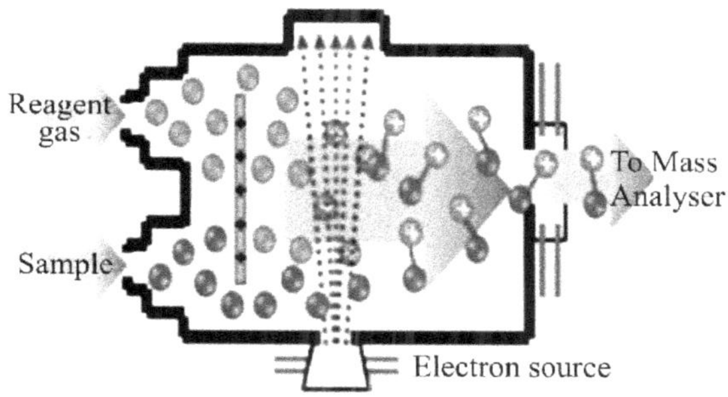

Fig.6.4 Chemical Ionization.
https://images.app.goo.gl/SU2wWpHXvzGYAGG18

Atmospheric Pressure Chemical Ionization: Identical to ESI interface. In APCI, the analyte is ionized in the atmospheric pressure area using a corona discharge. APCI's gas-phase ionization performs better than ESI when it comes to studying less-polar compounds. Methods like APCI and ESI complement each other. It is beneficial for less polar substances.

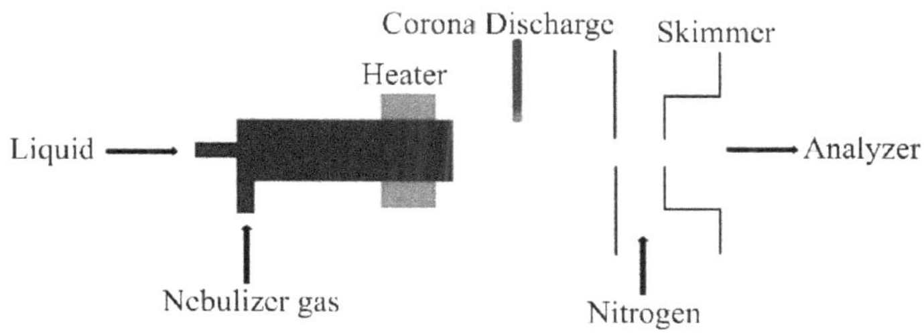

Fig.6.5 Atmospheric Pressure Chemical Ionization.
https://images.app.goo.gl/NPiGgNBgYpis1DBn9

2. Mass Analyzer:

Quadrupole Mass Analyzer: The quadrupole mass filter is the mass analyzer that is used the most frequently. Four solid rods with circular or hyperbolic cross sections that are evenly spaced apart and perpendicular to the ion route make up the quadrupole. Instead of using magnetic fields like the magnet-sector mass spectrometer does, the quadrupole uses electric fields to differentiate the ions according to their m/z. By applying a combination of radio frequency (RF) and direct-current (DC) voltages with the opposite polarity to each rod on the pairs of opposite rods, isolation is achieved. By adjusting the field strengths, it is possible to separate ions with stable oscillations from those with unstable oscillations, causing the former to strike a rod, become neutral, and then be drawn out of the analyzer by the vacuum system.

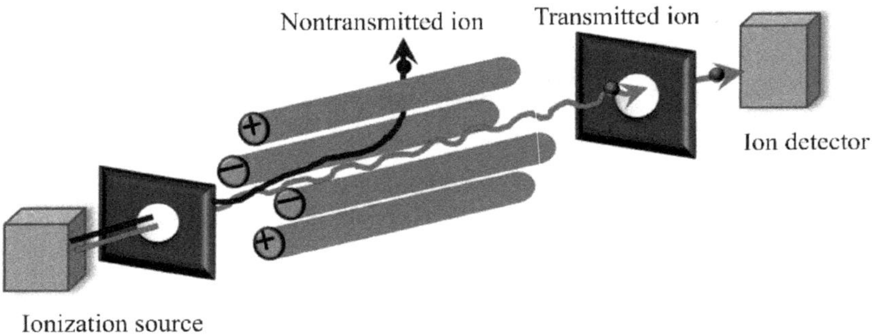

Fig.6.6 Quadrupole Mass Analyzer.
https://images.app.goo.gl/PQfLFviKz2HUebbk9

Time -of –Flight (TOF): In a time-of-flight (TOF) mass analyzer, all ions are simultaneously subjected to a uniform electromagnetic force, which accelerates them down a flight tube. The mass-to-charge ratios of the ions are calculated by their entry times since lighter ions travel more quickly and arrive at the detector first. Time-of-flight mass analyzers are capable of measuring a wide variety of masses with high precision.

Quadrupole mass analyzers have consistent unit mass resolution across the entire mass range, while newer models like magnetic sector and ToF analyzer vary in mass resolution, with a resolving power defined as m/Δm for performance.

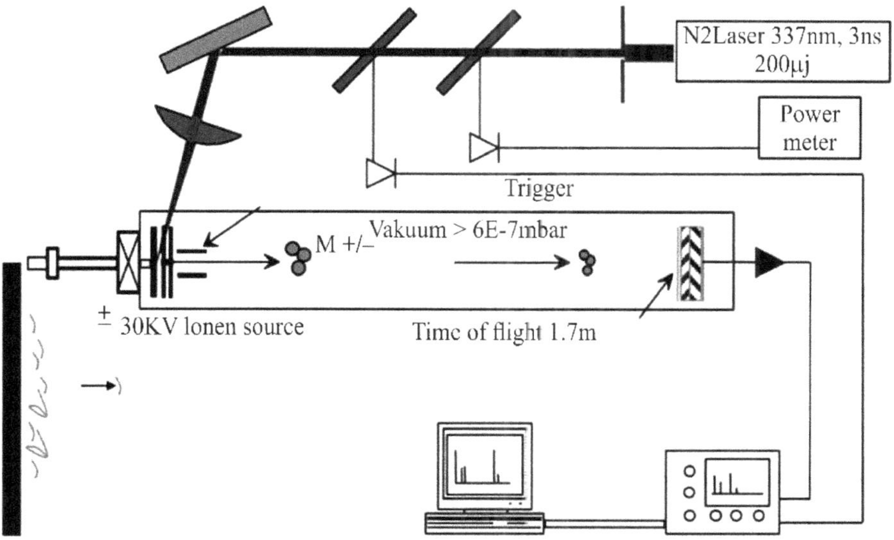

Fig.6.7 Time-of-Flight.
https://images.app.goo.gl/MgFB6dYzaGKLhNFV7

3. Vacuum System: High vacuum levels are necessary for mass analyzers to function dependably and accurately.

4. Detector: It is necessary to detect and turn the ion beam from the mass analyzer into a signal that may be used. The detector is a crucial component of the mass spectrometer that produces a signal from incident ions by either inducing a current (created by moving charges) or by producing secondary electrons, which are then amplified.

Mostly used detectors are Flame ionization detector, Thermal conductivity detector etc.

Advantages of GC-MS:

- High chromatographic resolution, sensitivity, and repeatability are all features of the GC-MC technology.
- Faster analysis, significantly expanded range of thermally labile and low volatility samples amenable to analysis
- Improved sensitivity, especially for compounds that are difficult to analyze and improve confidence in sample identification

- Structural determination of unknown organic compounds in complex mixtures by corresponding their spectra with reference spectra and by predetermined spectral interpretation.
- Used in quality control of industrial products.
- GC-MS is more affordable than LC-MS.
- Helium gas can survive for several months in a tank.

Disadvantages of GC-MS:

- Gas chromatography mass spectrometry (GC-MS) is limited to substances with vapor pressures above 10 torr, but can be examined at lower pressures for chemically derivatized substances. Positional substitution on aromatic rings can be challenging, and isomeric chemicals like naphthalene and azulene cannot be differentiated.
- *Accuracy limits*: The broad restrictions mentioned above have an impact on qualitative accuracy. The analytical process's calibration regulates quantitative correctness, with a normal accuracy of 20% relative standard deviation when using internal isotopic standards.
- The sensitivity and detection limits of an extract with 0.1 to 100 ng of each component may be required, depending on the dilution factor and ionization method.

Applications of GC-MS:

1. **Analysis of food, drinks and perfumes:** GC-MS is commonly used to analyze sweet-smelling intensifiers in nourishments and refreshes, including unsaturated fats, alcohols, aldehydes, and terpenes, which are naturally present or added during treatment.
2. **Environmental monitoring:** GC-MS is a highly recommended technology for environmental monitoring, offering cost-effective and reliable equipment for screening organic compounds like pesticides, herbicides in soil and water and sulphur in air.
3. **Biological determinations:** In order to check for the presence of anesthetics, drugs, alcohols, residual solvents, and other medications like anticonvulsants and barbiturates in blood and urine, only GC-MS is utilized.
4. **DOP analysis:** The primary tool used in anti-doping laboratories in sports is the GC-MS, which is used to check competitors' pee samples for banned performance-enhancing drugs like anabolic steroids.
5. **Forensic analysis:** GC-MS can look at body component particles to help link a criminal to a transgression.

6. **Pesticide determination:** Pesticide determination using GC-MS involves extracting pesticides from samples and derivatizing them for better analysis. The pesticides are then separated using Gas Chromatography (GC) and detected using Mass Spectrometry (MS).

   The pesticides are identified by matching their retention times and mass spectra with known standards. Quantification is done using calibration curves and internal standards to ensure accurate results.

   GC-MS techniques like Selected Ion Monitoring (SIM) and Multiple Reaction Monitoring (MRM) are used for targeted and sensitive detection. Scan Mode is used for identifying unknown pesticides.

   The GC-MS method is validated and quality-checked to ensure accuracy, precision, and sensitivity.

7. **Phytoconstituents determination:** The extracted extract was analyzed using GC-MS, which is helpful for figuring out the amount of the active ingredients in herbal plants are employed in cosmetics, medications, food, and pharmaceutical sectors.

   Also used for the determination of alkaloids, terpenoids, glycosides and flavonoids.

8. **Industrial purposes:** The examination of aromatic solvents, inorganic gases, amino alcohol in water, contaminants in styrene, glycol, diols, xylene, allergies in cosmetics, and other materials is done in industries using GC-MS.

   Formic acid in acetic acid is characterized using GC-MS for industrial applications.

9. **Reasearch purposes:** A unique chance to analyze novel compounds for characterisation and identification of synthesized or derivatized compounds is presented by GC-MS. It is extensively employed in both pure and practical sciences, including biotechnology, chemistry, polymers, and nanotechnology.

10. **Toxicity in clinical situations:** By using GC-MS, the toxin and venoms are detected.

11. **Protection and detection of chemical warfare agents:** An integral component of a chemical analysis unit is the GC-MS and for improving preparation for public health and homeland security.

12. **Geochemical investigations:** GC-MS is useful for organic geoscience applications because of its significantly increased molecular ions, substantial isomer and structurally relevant mass spectrum peaks, broader range of low-volatile hydrocarbons that are accessible to investigation, and unique isotope ratio information.

References

1. ASHISH C, Manish Kumar. G and Priyanka .C, GC-MS Technique and its Analytical Applications in Science and Technology, Journal of Analytical & Bioanalytical Technique, November 2014
2. Hearn, Ionization Methods in Organic Mass Spectrometry, UK College of Arts and Science
3. Komal P, Poournima. S,Dr. Sachin .P, Pranali. P, Ashwini.P, Prathamesh.S, Applications of GC-MS Used In Herbal Plants , International Journal of Pharmaceutical Research and Applications, May - June 2021 Volume 6, Issue 3,pp:1193-1196
4. Riya. U, Khyati .P, Dr Umesh. U, A Review Article on Advancements in GC-MS Gas Chromatography – Mass Spectrometry (GC–MS), International Journal of Pharmaceutical Research and Applications, Mar-Apr 2023, Volume 8, Issue 2
5. S. Z. Hussain, Khushnuma Maqbool, GC-MS: Principle, Technique and its application in Food Science, International Journal of Current Science, 2014, No. No.13, 116-126 ref. 33
6. Willard, Merritt, Dean, Settle, Instrumental Methods of Analysis, sixth edition.

Questions

1. Enlist the components used in the GC-MS instrumentation.
2. Why interface used in this hyphenated technique?
3. What is the limitation of time- of- light analyzer?
4. What interfaces used in the GC-MS?
5. Write a note on jet /orifice interface.
6. Difference between EI and ESI.

CHAPTER 7

Gas Chromatography-Nuclear Magnetic Resonance (GC-NMR)

Introduction

The 1960s marked the introduction of the GC-NMR method. Initially, an NMR (nuclear magnetic resonance) glass microtube was filled with the separated components of the sample from gas chromatography (GC) using a syringe. Flow cell NMR tubes were added to the GCNMR system in the 1970s to enable the input of separated sample components from GC into NMR. Buddrus and Hertzog presented the first GC-NMR hyphenated technique in 1980, despite the fact that these two were not truly hyphenated techniques. GC and NMR were connected using an NMR tube that was shaped like a flow cell with both sides open. Many developments came after, including the introduction of the on-flow and stop-flow modes.

Principle: This method combines the NMR with the GC. Component identification is carried out by NMR, and component separation is accomplished by GC. This technique's hyphenation gives the molecules structural details of the fragmented components.

Instrumentation: The main components of GC-NMR include:

1. GC unit
2. NMR unit

1. GC unit:

(i) Carrier gas: Gas chromatography uses He, Ar, and N_2 as mobile phases, which are inert gases that don't react with the sample or stationary phase. The choice of carrier gas depends on the instrument's detector requirements. Flow rates for packed and capillary columns vary between 25-150 mL/min and 1-25 mL/min, depending on column type.

(ii) Flow regulators and flow meters: Use a Rota meter or a Soap bubble flow meter to provide the gas at a consistent pressure and flow rate.

Rota meters: Positioned prior to column intakes, they have a glass tube with a float secured by a spring. The pace at which carrier gas flows controls the float's level.

***Soap Bubble Meter*:** Works similarly to a Rota meter, except instead of a float, the flow rate is shown by a soap bubble that forms.

(iii) Injectors: The septum that makes up the injection port is where the syringe needle is inserted to inject the sample.

Using a tiny syringe, the sample is often injected into an inert gas stream at a high temperature.

The stationary phase is placed into a column together with the vaporized sample.

There are many injection devices available they are:

(a) Split mode: The sample is injected through a rubber septum using a microliter syringe, mixed with carrier gas in a glass liner, and a small fraction enters the capillary column, while the rest exits through a split vent. The flow rate can be controlled to control the sample fraction.

(b) Splitless mode: The split vent is closed, allowing all carrier gas to enter the column, enabling splitless injection for trace analysis. However, low flow rate through the injector can cause precolumn band widening. The solvent condenses at the capillary column entrance, creating a barrier to trap solutes. The separation process begins when column temperature is raised following solute concentration.

(c) Large Volume on column injector: Using this technique, the sample is injected straight—that is, without heating—into the column. After that, the temperature in the column is raised, volatilizing the sample at the lowest feasible temperature.

(iv) Column: One of the crucial components of GC that determines the effectiveness of separation is the column. Stainless steel and glass are used to make columns.

This is the location of the sample's chromatographic separation.

There are several kinds of columns available for various chromatographic uses.

Chromatographic columns are divided into two main categories: packed and capillary.

Packed columns handle larger samples, while capillary columns separate complex mixes. Capillaries, made of fused silica, are covered in a polymer for protection. They range in length from 15 to 100 meters and have an interior diameter of 150 to 300 micrometers.

There are three main types of capillary columns: wall-coated open tubular columns (WCOT), porous-layer open tubular columns (PLOT), and open tubular columns with support coating (SCOT).

Each type has a different coating of stationary phase on the inner wall.

2. NMR unit:

(i) **Magnet:** A magnetic field is produced when these coils are subjected to an electric current. The sample's atomic nuclei are in contact with the magnetic field of the coils.

(ii) **Permanent Magnet:** Within the NMR device, a permanent magnet produces a consistent magnetic field. Typically, the magnetic field intensity falls between 60 and 100 MHz.

(iii) **Sweep Generator:** The sweep generator modifies the sample's magnetic field's strength. It allows adjustments and adjustments to ensure that the required magnetic field intensity is reached.

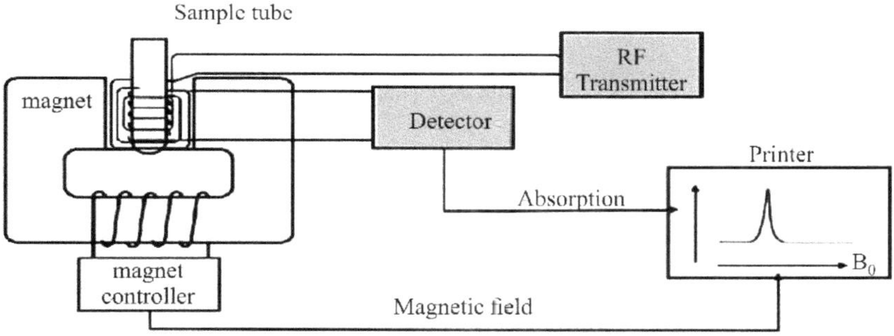

Fig. 7.1 Instrumentation of NMR unit.
https://images.app.goo.gl/FnJtNE2EDpRmurj68

(iv) **Radiofrequency Transmitter:** This part consists of a coil that pulses radio waves loudly and briefly. A radiofrequency pulse is applied to the sample in order to activate the atomic nuclei.

(v) **Radiofrequency Receiver:** As atomic nuclei relax to a lower energy level, radio frequencies are emitted. The radiofrequency receiver coil picks them up. It captures the NMR signals that the substance produces.

(vi) **RF Detector:** After the sample has been activated, the RF detector helps identify the unabsorbed radio frequencies. It provides details on the resonance frequencies and intensities of the NMR signals.

(vii) **Recorder:** A recorder captures the NMR signals that the RF detector receives. It gathers and stores information for further research.

Disadvantages

The issue with combining these two techniques is that materials utilized for analysis in GC are in a gaseous condition, but samples used for NMR investigation are liquid or solid. When using a carrier gas for NMR analysis, the signal acquired at atmospheric pressure will have a poor signal-to-noise ratio.

Applications

1. The most effective spectroscopic elucidation of the structures of unknown substances is obtained by combining GC with capillary NMR.
2. GC-NMR can distinguish between configurational and constitutional isomers. The same spectra are seen by enantiomers at varying retention times.
3. Used to determine the stereoisomers in a complicated combination

References

1. NMR-Spectroscopy – Definition, Principle, Steps, Parts, Uses; Microbiology notes; June 2023
2. Pallavi. P, Shilpa .K, Review on Hyphenated Techniques, International Journal of Chemical Studies, ISSN: 2321-4902 Volume 1 Issue 3
3. J S. Zavahir, Y. Nolvachai, and Philip J. Marriott, Molecular spectroscopy-Information rich 3 detection for gas chromatography
4. Nasrullah Shah, Muhammad Balal Arain and Mustafa .S, Historical background: milestones in the field of development of analytical instrumentation
5. David .H, Introduction to Gas Chromatography Instrumentation, Library texts chemistry

Questions

1. Discuss the disadvantages of GC-NMR.
2. Explain the instrumentation of GC-NMR.

CHAPTER 8

Gas Chromatography-Fourier Transform Infrared Spectroscopy (GC-FTIR)

Introduction

The two-phase method known as GC-FTIR (gas chromatography/Fourier transform infrared spectroscopy) uses the GC step to separate the specimens and the IR phase to identify them. A capillary-type GC columns is usually used to improve chromatography efficiency, and the infrared (IR) stage often consists of an interferometric (Fourier transformation or FT) spectroscopy. GC-FTIR can also produce findings that are quantitative, even though it is often employed to provide data that is qualitative on different kinds of the analytes.

Sophisticated GC-FTIR equipment can be used to separate complicated combinations of volatile materials while also allowing for the chemical characterization of the parts. Their functional categories can be determined via IR spectroscopy. The software for searching and building spectral libraries is accessible. The recognition of fractions could be spontaneous.

Principle: The GC-FTIR method operates according to the following principle: After the sample has been divided by gas chromatography each fraction reaches the interface with the instrument as a result of retention time. The interferometer-modified interference light settles on the interface's surface simultaneously. The reflected light is preferentially absorbed by every part in the interface, and the sensor subsequently picks up the resulting interfering signal. The computing system retains all of the interferogram data that was gathered from the sensor and uses a quick Fourier transform in order to get the individual gases' infrared spectrum. Finally, the database can be used to retrieve the molecular characteristics of each element.

Instrumentation:

Components of GC-FTIR:

- Carrier gas
- Injection system
- Column
- Oven
- Interfaces
- Interferogram
- Detector

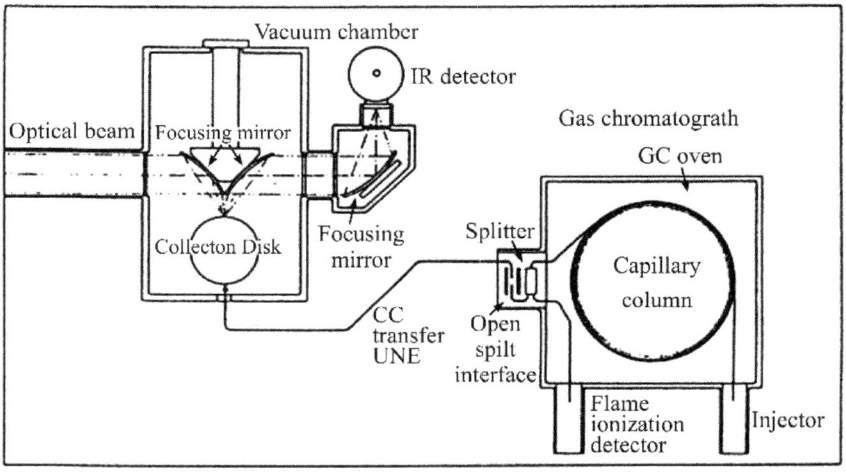

Fig. 8.1 Instrumentation of GC-FTIR.
www.sciencedirect.com/science/article/abs/pii/S0165993602008129

- **Carrier gas:** The carrier gas, or mobile phase, must be chemically inert and is commonly placed in pressurized tanks. The flow rate is regulated by pressure regulators, gauges, and flow meters, with typical flow rates for packed columns being 25-150 mL/min and 1–25 mL/min for open tubular capillary columns.

  The most widely utilized gas is helium, although argon, nitrogen, and hydrogen are also employed.

- **Injection system:** Samples are inserted as vapor plugs, injected into a heated sample port at 50°C beyond boiling point, and transported to the column using calibrated micro syringes, ensuring proper temperature control.

- **Column:** Gas chromatography involves sample components traveling through capillary columns coated with stationary phase or silicon particles, typically several meters long (10-120m) or inner diameter (0.10-0.50 mm), compared to packed columns with a diameter of 2-4 mm and length(1-5m).

- **Oven:** The temperature of the gas chromatographic ovens, which are configurable for temperature, normally ranges from 5℃ to 400℃ but can go as low as -25℃ with cryogenic cooling.
- **Interface:** An essential component of the integrated device is the connection in GC-FTIR. There are now two different types of industrial interfaces: frozen trap interface and light pipe interface. Although the frozen recording interface has a low detection limit and a large ratio of signal to noise, it is costly and challenging to use. Real-time documentation, cheapness, and ease of use are all benefits provided by the currently commonly employed light pipe connection.

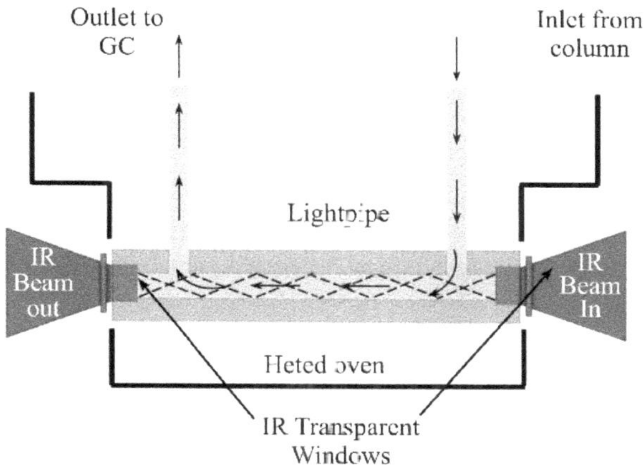

Fig. 8.2 Light Pipe Interface.
https://images.app.goo.gl/tw6k3j4ao7afq2di9

Fiberglass tube with gold coating is the Light pipe (LP). The entire optical efficiency of the cell is enhanced by the presence of a gold covering by permitting numerous reflections of the IR light. This substance is regarded as being extraordinarily powerful, stable, and inert to chemicals, which is a big plus for a substance that requires heating and has to be analytically inert. By the reverse hand, the extremely high temperature of the LP becomes an issue since it causes a rapid decrease in the level of the signal.

The heated LP, being constitutes an IR reflector within and of themselves, emits an immense quantity of unmodulated infrared light that consumes the detector's filter or amplifier and causes this to happen. By adding a cold barrier to the conclusion of the hot LP, the objective becomes pointless.

- **Interferogram:**

A rapid-scanning two-beam FTIR instrument delivers the modified IR channel to a piece of FTIR equipment connected to a gas chromatograph (GC), which is effectively a single-beam FTIR spectrometer. An interferometer that often follows the initial Michelson design. An IR stream of energy can be divided into two distinct channels using the Michelson interferometer device. It was first presented by two beams divided by a light-splitter, then afterwards, following the path difference, by one modulated light moving reflector. As a result, an IR sensor may measure variations in intensity among these as an effect of route variation, structure, and the interferometer's disruption pattern, or interferogram.

It's the Fourier transform's polar opposite in terms of theme. Rapid-scanning interferometers usually work by doing a series of images resulting in an average the data. Each interferogram requires a specific rate of sampling in order to combine the signals accurately. a constant pause after each scan. As a result, it's crucial to very precisely align the adjustable mirrors to control the path of light difference's irregular behaviour.

- **Detector:**

Intensity is one of the primary issues in the GC/FTIR investigation because the vast majority of common GC detectors (flame ionization, capturing electrons, mass spectroscopy, an alkaline flame, and more) have limits on detection between one and five orders in magnitude less than FTIR. The recommended detector is the mercury and cadmium telluride (MCT) detector. According on the spectral assortment, this detector increases S/N by a factor of 5 to 50 comparing to the usual triglycine sulphate (TGS) detectors.

In infrared (FTIR) spectroscopy, the MCT detector is a specific kind of quantum detector. Due to its outstanding sensitivity, it is used over substitute detectors in gas chromatography-FTIR (GC-FTIR) studies.

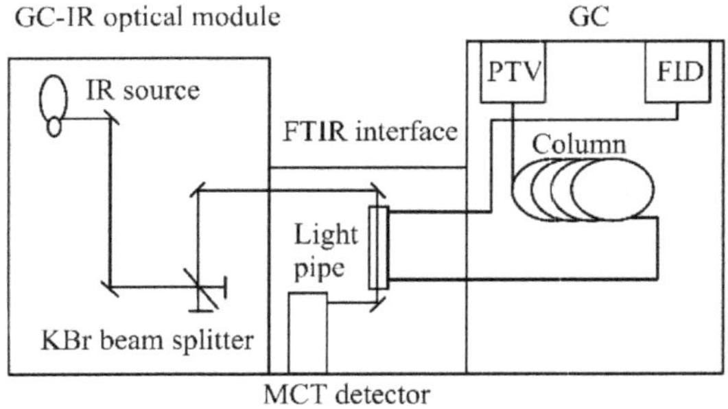

Fig. 8.3 MCT Detector.

www.sciencedirect.com/topics/earth-and-planetary-sciences/mercury-cadmium-telluride

In GC-FTIR, a collimated light beam generated by the spectrometer is used to install the MCT detector on the opposite side of the FTIR. It has an embedded 120mm long, 1.0 mm i.d.43 light pipe. The stainless-steel detector has a high-sensitivity MCT-A (with a range 11,700 to 600cm -1) that is recommended.

The waste product from the GC flows via a warmed transferring line with the composition of gas before reaching the light pipe via an electronically GC/FTIR coupling mechanism. Throughout an examination, the interferograms are continuously examined (an average of one image per sec). This enables the calculation of only one beam's IR Spectroscopy using the Fourier transform and the Gram-Schmidt vector method, measuring time, as well as the immediate reconstructing of a chromatogram. This is evaluated in relation to a spectrum that was collected prior to the material being put inside the GC. The program corresponds, co-adds, and separates the spectrum for each GC peak once the real run is finished.

The most accurate IR spectra are generated when one GC peak fills a light pipe, ensuring a single peak travel through without crossing over others. The constituent pressure of gases must align with the light-pipe capacity via the GC column. Sensitivity depends on the temperature of the light-pipe, as an example, a make-up gas is required.

Advantages of GC-FTIR:

- Gas chromatography-Fourier transform infrared spectroscopy (GC-FTIR) is a powerful analytical method that combines gas chromatography's high-efficiency separation capabilities with molecular structure identification.
- It allows real-time measurements and has a large library of gas phase IR spectra for searching for GC elutes. GC-FTIR can speed up the identification of functional groups in unidentified substances, supplementing mass spectrometry's information.
- High sensitivity: GC-FTIR is capable of detecting traces of substances in complicated combinations.
- Good selectivity: GC-FTIR can distinguish among substances having related structural features.
- GC-FTIR also provides additional data in addition to mass spectrometry (MS) and NMR, two commonly used analysis methods.

Disadvantages:

- GC-FTIR spectroscopy are vapor phase bands and are very dissimilar from condensed phase spectroscopy.
- There are numerous data collecting and reporting options that can be accomplished using software programs. Rotating fine structure

features that are frequently stretched out in both solids and liquids are frequently observed in vaporized state spectra.

- Vapor phase also lacks highly informative bands that are present in the compressed phase because of interactions between molecules (H-bonding). However, a variety of computerized information bases for steam phase spectrum are now accessible.

Applications:

- **Environmental**:

  GC/IR has been used to analyze environmental contaminants qualitatively and quantitatively, offering advantages such as precision, selection, isomer differentiation, and early realization of complementary characteristics. Initiatives to enhance GC/FTIR interactions, particularly the LP interface, have been motivated by environmental concerns. This approach provides minimum detectable concentrations for standards, soil samples, and herbicides, and has proven quantitative skills for priority pollutants.

- **Flavour and fragrance:**

  GC/IR is mostly used to identify flavour and aroma components. For volatile flavouring compounds, the mutually beneficial properties of GC/IR for structure investigation were recognized accurately early. concentrating especially on IR's specific ability Individual isomers can be distinguished using spectrophotometer.

- **Fatty acids:**

  To determine the total quantity of trans fatty acids in foods and to discriminate among Cis soluble Trans isomers in petroleum and fats, IR spectroscopy is used. Each isomer in a combination of unsaturated fat complexes can be examined in the infrared using GC/FTIR technology. In the first instance, heated oils were used to create separated conjugated cyclical fatty acid combinations utilizing an LP connection. However, the sensitivity of HRGC equipment is higher for detecting minor components in mixtures with uneven concentration ranges, including trans Polyunsaturated levels. It is also possible to investigate complex fatty acid combinations using the double-sided interface.

- **Pesticide analysis:**

  In pesticides chemical research, GC/FTIR is used to monitor responses over time and define the ideal amounts of targeted products. The ideal ratios are determined by regularly collecting aliquot information regarding response materials.

- **Quantitative analysis of caffeine:**

  Actual spectrum frame chromatography is used to determine the correct caffeine amounts for quantitative evaluation. Caffeine's largest peak ranges from 1650 and 1700 cm-1, whereas diphenylamine's maximum area is around 1475 and 1525 cm-1. For 6 concentrations of substances, the relationship coefficient is 0.997. This method aids in figuring out the amount of caffeine exists in coffee and samples of urine.

- **Compositional studies of high temperature coal tar:**

  The residue of cooking procedures called coal tar is essential in both industrial and ecological uses. fortunately, because of the different charcoal and heating circumstances, its composition is still unclear. To identify the different isomers in coal tar, scientists are utilizing capillaries GC/FTIR as well as retention indices (RIs).

- **Other applications**:

  Used in analysis of perfumes

  Used in analysis of spirit

  Used in analysis of unknown illicit drugs

References

1. Instrumental methods of chemical analysis by H. Kuar, Pragati prakashan, 4th edition, January 2012.
2. Original research article, Front. Chem., 24 July 2020, Sec. Analytical Chemistry Volume 8 – 2020
3. P. M. Phole, Applications of GC-FTIR in Pharmaceutical Analysis, International Journal of Pharmaceutical Research and Applications, Volume 7, Issue 4 July-Aug 2022, pages 1133-1140
4. Tom Visser, FT-IR detection in gas chromatography, Trends in Analytical Chemistry, Volume 21, Issues 9–10, 10 September 2002, Pages 627-636

Questions

1. Write a note on applications of GC-FTIR.
2. Add a note on interfaces and working of GC-FTIR with neat labelled diagram.
3. Write a note instrumentation, advantages and disadvantages of GC-FTIR.

CHAPTER 9

Gas Chromatography- Atomic Absorption Spectroscopy (GC-AAS)

Introduction

Hyphenated technology is an efficient method for studying element forms, combining the selectivity and sensitivity of atomic absorption spectrometry with the high separation efficiency of chromatograms.

The benefits of gas chromatography (GC) are its straightforward operation, high separation efficiency, quick analytical speed, and little sample consumption. It is extensively employed in the analysis and separation of volatile materials. Morphological study of complicated mixtures comprising metals and certain non-metal elements may be carried out using GC-AAS technology. The gaseous components that have been separated by gas chromatography as well as the carrier gas can be immediately introduced into the atomic spectrum for direct examination and determination using GC-AAS technology.

Principle: In GC-AAS, the material is initially separated using gas chromatography before arriving at the AA system. Light may be absorbed by any atom or ion at a particular wavelength. The only particles in the sample that will absorb light at the characteristic wavelength are the atoms or ions of the analyte of interest. The concentration of the absorbing atoms or ions is directly proportional to the amount of light absorbed at this wavelength.

Instrumentation:

The components of GC-AAS are:

1. Gas chromatography
   - (i) Carrier gas
   - (ii) Flow regulators and flow meters
   - (iii) Injection devices
   - (iv) Columns

2. Interface
3. AAS
   - (i) Light source
   - (ii) Atomizer
   - (iii) Monochromators
   - (iv) Detector

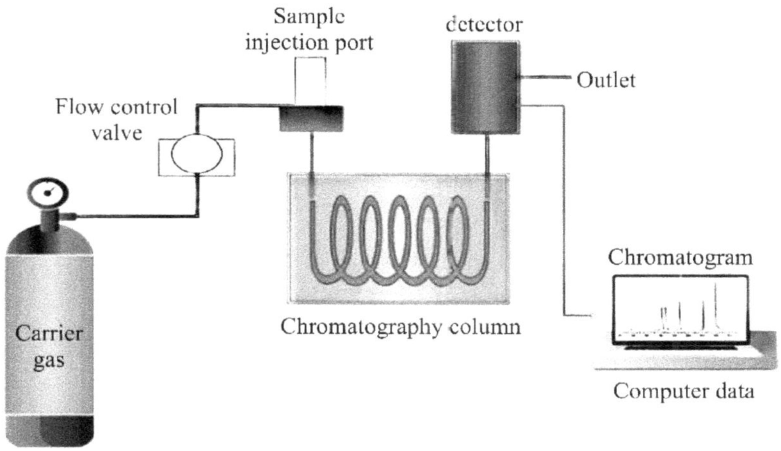

Fig.9.1 Instrumentation of GC.
https://images.app.goo.gl/SdrzHNxyTKL2sJ3C7

1. Gas chromatography:

(i) Carrier gas:

The carrier gas, which differs depending on the GC being utilized, is crucial. The carrier gas used in gas chromatography needs to be dry, oxygen-free, and chemically inert. Because it is safer than hydrogen but comparable in efficiency, has a wider range of flow rates, and works with a variety of detectors, helium is employed most frequently. Depending on the intended performance and the detector being utilized, nitrogen, argon, and hydrogen are also employed.

(ii) Flow regulators and flow meters:

Use a Rota meter or a Soap bubble flow meter to provide the gas at a consistent pressure and flow rate.

***Rota meters*:** positioned prior to column intakes, they have a glass tube with a float secured by a spring. The pace at which carrier gas flows controls the float's level.

Soap Bubble Meter: Works similarly to a Rota meter, except instead of a float, the flow rate is shown by a soap bubble that forms.

(iii) Injection devices:

The septum that makes up the injection port is where the syringe needle is inserted to inject the sample.

Using a tiny syringe, the sample is often injected into an inert gas stream at a high temperature.

The stationary phase is placed into a column together with the vaporized sample.

To guarantee quick and thorough solute volatilization, the injector's temperature should be between 30 and 50 degrees Celsius higher than the column temperature. The septum that makes up the injection port is where a syringe needle is placed to inject the sample

The port for injection is a heated, glass-lined, hollow cylinder:

To ensure that every element in the sample vaporizes, the injector is heated.

Overheating the injection temperature might cause the specimen to break down or alter structurally.

There are many injection devices available they are:

(a) Split mode

(b) Splitless mode

(c) Large Volume on column injector

(iv) Columns:

One of the crucial components of GC that determines the effectiveness of separation is the column. Stainless steel and glass are used to make columns.

This is the location of the sample's chromatographic separation.

There are several kinds of columns available for various chromatographic uses.

The system's central component.

It has a stationary phase coating on it, which significantly affects how the chemicals separate.

Column types vary depending on their nature.

Packed columns are commercially available in non-polar to polar configurations.

Open tubular/capillary columns are made of long capillary tubing (30-90 meters) with a diameter of 0.025 to 0.075 cm, made of stainless steel. They are coil-shaped and coated with stationary phase liquid in the form of a thin film on the inner wall.

2. Interface:

To serve as an optical table for the magnetically installed optical components of the A.A., an eighth-inch steel plate was positioned atop the G.C. To facilitate the passage of the transfer line and its heater, a hole with a diameter of 1/2 inch was bored through the plate. A stainless steel transfer line served as the direct link between the G.C. and the lower electrode. A teflon ferrule, which also functioned as an electrical isolation device, sealed the transfer line to the electrode. To track the temperature of the transfer line, a chromel-alumel thermocouple pyrometer was employed. Pyrex capillary tubing was eventually used to replace the stainless steel transfer line.

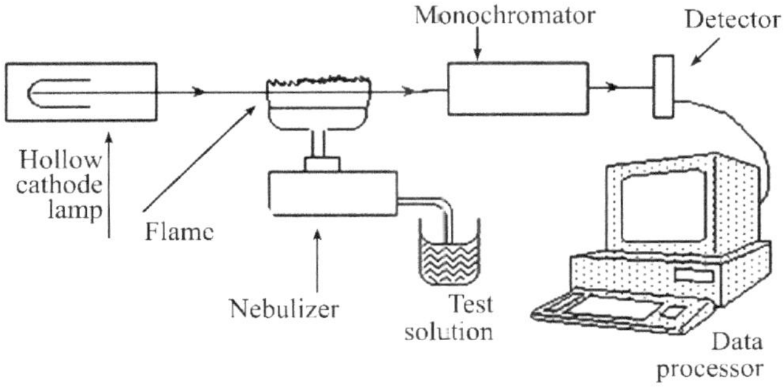

Fig.9.2 Instrumentation of AAS.

https://images.app.goo.gl/5F4a83wUk4JEwzkWA

3. AAS:

(i) Light source:

Hallow cathode lamp:

For the majority of elements that can be determined by atomic absorption, the hollow cathode lamp provides a very good, brilliant line source. Often, a hollowed-out cylinder made of the metal in which the spectrum is to be generated serves as the lamp's cathode. A glass cylinder that is often partially filled with argon or neon at low pressure houses the sealed anode and cathode. A window that is transparent to the radiation released is located at the end of the glass cylinder.

A portion of the fill gas atoms ionize when an electrical potential is placed between the anode and cathode. The process known as "sputtering" occurs when the positively charged fill gas ions speed across the electrical field, colliding with the negatively charged cathode and displacing individual metal atoms. Then, by impacting with fill gas ions, spewed metal atoms are stimulated to an emission state by a kinetic energy transfer.

The lifespan of hollow cathode lamps is limited.

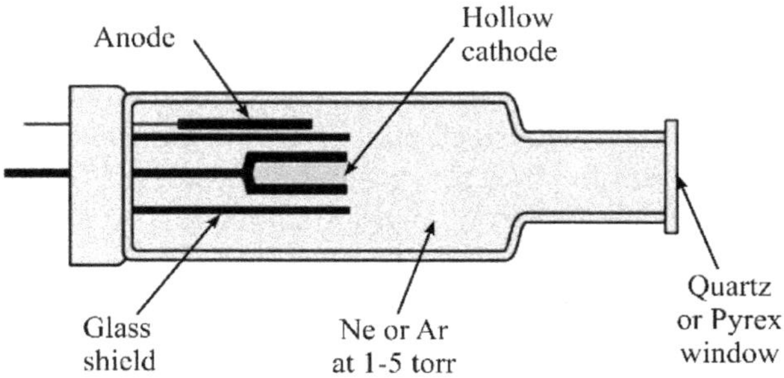

Fig.9.3 Hallow Cathode Lamp.
https://images.app.goo.gl/GDwQHvYqBauTtTBR7

Electrodeless discharge lamp:

Electrodeless discharge lamps (EDLs) use a quartz bulb sealed with a metal or salt source to create an RF field. This energy vaporizes and excites the atoms inside the bulb, emitting their characteristic spectrum. An accessory power supply is required to operate an EDL. EDLs are typically more intense and sensitive than hollow cathode lamps, offering better precision and lower detection limits in areas with limited intensity.

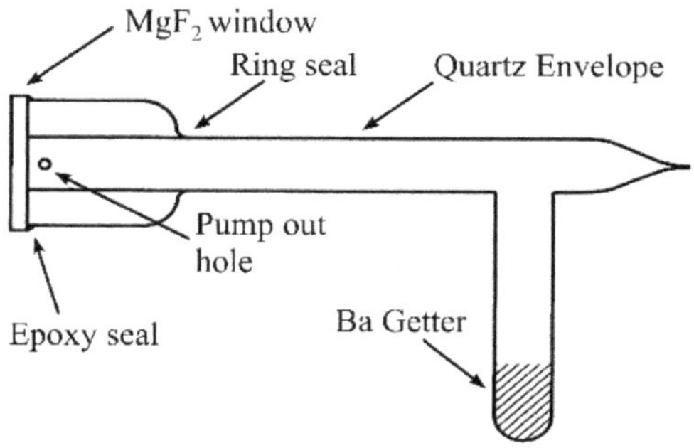

Fig.9.4 Electrodeless Discharge Lamp.
https://images.app.goo.gl/UkMHiUB63eDtSwQ9A

(ii) Atomizer:

Premix-up chamber:

The sample solution in this "premix" setup is sprayed into the mixing chamber as a fine aerosol after it has passed through a nebulizer.

Here, fuel and oxidant gases are combined with the sample aerosol before it is transported to the burner head, where burning and sample atomization take place.

Total consumption burner:

The burner is called total consumption as the entire sample is atomized in the flame.

Fuel, oxidizing gases, and sample solution enter through several passageways and come together at the flame aperture. The flame breaks the liquid sample into droplets, burning and evaporating, leaving a reduced remnant of atoms.

(iii) Monochromators:

The monochromator is a crucial component of an AA spectrophotometer, used to separate thousands of lines and filter out other wavelengths. It helps identify the sample's absorbable wavelength and filter out other wavelengths, enabling the identification of the chosen element even when others are present.

They come in two varieties:

***Monochromator prism*:** Prisms are made from quartz material because it is clear throughout.

***Grating monochromator*:** It is a planar surface with a number of parallel, straight lines cut into it.

(iv) Detectors:

The purpose of the detector, which is usually a photomultiplier tube, is to translate the light signal into an electrical signal proportionate to the light intensity. The monochromator selects the light that is focused upon it. An amplifier that processes signals is responsible for processing electrical signals. The signal might be supplied into a data station for output using the required format, or it could be displayed for reading.

Advantages:

- Morphological study of complicated mixtures comprising metals and certain non-metal elements may be carried out using GC-AAS technology.
- For direct analysis and determination, GC-AAS technology may enter the gaseous components separated by gas chromatography and the carrier gas directly into the atomic spectrum.
- It has high detection sensitivity and selectivity

Disadvantages:

- Low column efficiency, extremely long preconditioning time.
- Peak suppression while analyzing an actual sample.

Applications:

1. Environmental analysis:

- Examination of low-level pollutants
- Trace element levels in polluted soil are measured (soil analysis).
- Magnesium and calcium content analysis in tap water (water analysis).

2. Clinical analysis:

- Measuring the concentration of metals in biological fluids, including serum, urine, and blood.

3. Pharmaceuticals:

- The finished medications may include trace quantities of the catalyst employed. Consequently, the amount of catalyst present is determined using AAS.

4. Mining:

- The content of metal such as gold present in the rock can be determined.

5. Food analysis:

- The trace elements present in the food components can be detected.

6. Others:

- Lead content in paint can be analyzed.
- Trace metal monitoring in streams of industrial effluent.
- Examination of the purity in steels and other metal alloys.

References

1. Subham Kumar. V, GC-AAS (Gas Chromatography-Atomic Absorption spectrometry), Research gate, 2021.
2. Chromatography-Atomic Absorption Spectroscopy Technology, BOC Sciences
3. R. Dumarey, R. Dams, P. Sandra, Interfacing an atomic absorption spectrophotometer with a fused silica capillary gas chromatographic system for the determination of trace organomercury(II) compounds, Wiley online library.
4. Richard D. Beaty and Jack D. Kerber, Concepts, Instrumentation and Techniques in Atomic Absorption Spectrophotometry, The Perkin-Elmer Corporation, Second edition.
5. Eric Leon Kiesel, Development and Applications of Gas Chromatography - Atomic Absorption Interface Instrumentation, Louisiana State University

Questions

1. Write the applications of GC-AAS.
2. Mention the principle involved in GC-AAS.
3. Explain the instrumentation of GC-AAS.

CHAPTER 10

Fourier Transform (FT) NMR Spectroscopy (FT-NMR)

Introduction

Fourier-transform Radiofrequency, or RF, radiation pulses are used by NMR instruments to trigger magnetic field nuclei to turn into a higher-energy configuration. The frequency range of the RF pulse (usually 1–10 s) is sufficient to simultaneously activate nuclei in all local surroundings because of the Heisenberg uncertainty concept. A free-induction decay (FID) is a pattern of interference in the resulting RF output versus time that results from all of the nuclei reemitting RF radiation at their individual resonance frequencies. A Fourier transformation of the time-dependent data is used to separate the frequencies from their FID.

Principle: (FT-NMR) is a potent analytical method used to investigate the molecular structure. The fundamental idea that supports NMR is that when subjected to an external electromagnetic field, specific nuclei exist in particular nuclear spin states. The transitions between these various spin states that are unique to the specific nuclei in issue, as well as the chemical surroundings of that nuclei, are seen by NMR.

The fundamental mathematical operation required to transform data from the time domain (interferogram) to the frequency range (NMR spectrum) is known as the Fourier Transformation. The Spectrometer Frequency, Wave Width, Absorption Time, the number of Points, and Sweep Width are the most crucial variables that influence every spectrum you may acquire using an FT-NMR spectroscopy.

Instrumentation of FT-NMR:

Components Of FT-NMR:

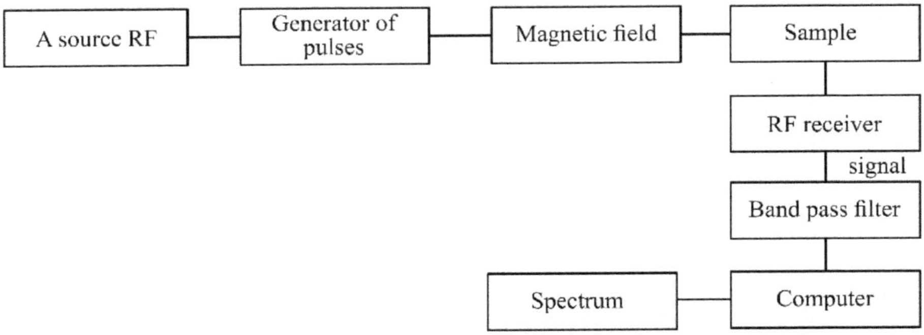

1. The radio emitter coil which emits a brief, strong electromagnetic pulse.
2. A strong magnet that generates tremendous fields of magnetism.
3. To ensure that the test component is exposed to a consistent magnetic force, the sample is put into a tube made of glass which rotates.
4. A receiver for radio wire that picks up radio waves released as nuclei drop their electrical charge.
5. A computing device that records and analyses data.
6. In the Fourier transform NMR devices, a hollow tube spins around the vertical z-axis and is inserted into the hole of a magnetic field or a motor.

FT- NMR INSTRUMENTATION

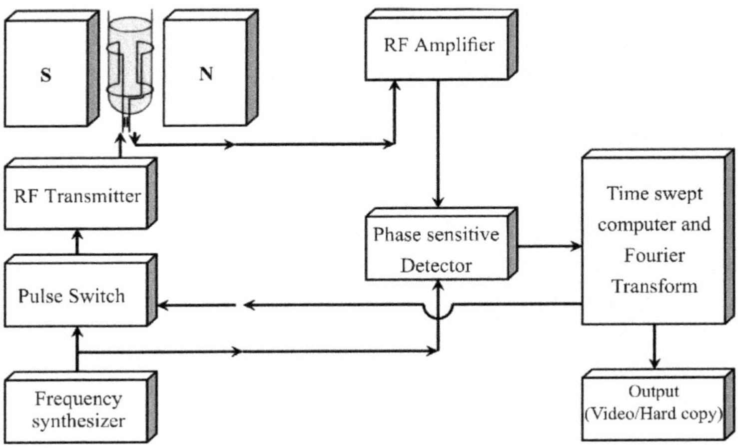

Fig.10.1 Instrumentation of FT-NMR.
https://images.app.goo.gl/x3uYU5QEQf19PnFA8

1. **Sample Stimulation**
   - **(i) Power of the RF pulse:** In pulse NMR, the amount of energy of the RF pulse utilized for stimulation determines the strength of the signal observed. The Magnetization rotates by a 90° pulse when the RF strength and pulse width are appropriate. A relaxing process takes place. The magnetization's strength diminishes gradually. The signal that results has been referred as Free Induction Decay (FID).
   - **(ii) Pulse duration and recycling time:** All precessional frequency that fall into the pulse's active range are stimulated. In the temporal area, the magnitude is inversely related to the pulse frequency. The pulse is stronger the wider the pulse's spectral area.
2. **Detector:** Recognizes the decrease of magnetism over time. A straightforward rapidly falling sine waves is the FID that corresponds to the absorbed energy of a single spectrum of frequencies. The FID is made up of a number of overlapping wave forms as well as noise and is modulated by all of the wavelengths. FID including time is referred to as a temporal phase spectrum.

   Other factors:
   1. Percentage uniformity
   2. The electromagnetic field's constancy
   3. The item being tested contains paramagnetic components.
   4. Heterogeneous nuclei transfer
3. **Digitization**: Digitized using an ADC (analogue to digital converter). It is stored on a computer as a collection of integers. The time difference ($\triangle$t) between sampling locations for the FID. It displays the highest rate that the FID is capable of measuring.

   $$\text{Specular width (Sw)} = 1/2 \times \triangle t.$$

   Evaluates how well a device can discriminate among signals and electrical noise

   $$S/N = \text{Mean/Standard deviation}$$

   It depends on factors including the sample's characteristics and the tool being used. The magnitude of the induced field of magnets affects the S/N ratio.

   $$S/N \text{ is directly proportional to } [H_0]^{3/2}$$

   S/N will improve with increasing the field's magnetic strength.

   S/N = Output amplitude average/root mean squaring (RMS) noise.

   RMS noise is equal to the median of peak-to-peak sound (2.5)

Signal to noise ratio (S/N) enhancement

S/N strengthening is necessary for PMR spectra when there are minute amounts of material. Since NMR experiments might have extremely low sensitivity, augmentation is frequently used in NMR studies on additional nuclei.

1. Suitably designed instruments
2. Averaged signal to separate signal from noise.
3. By FT employing filtering methods.

Advantages of FT-NMR:

The powerful analytical method known as FT-NMR has a number of benefits over the use of continuous wave NMR.

- **Time saving:** FT-NMR can simultaneously scan all NMR-active protons in a molecule, giving samples with nuclei other than 1H better structural information.
- **Greater sensitivity:** By combining spectrum responses over a specified time period, signal-to-noise ratios are enhanced, resulting in greater sensitivity.
- **More sensitivity for research on other nuclei:** Due to signal averaging, FT-NMR offers more sensitive for studies on different nuclei including 13C, 31P, and 19F compared to CW-NMR, which is predominantly employed for 1H investigations.
- **Exceptional improvement in sensitivity:** This frequently yields informative data from the small sample sizes available.
- With a minimum of 5mg of the substance, FT-NMR can be obtained.
- The signals are distinct and there is very little electrical background noise present.
- Additionally, the field of engineering, commercial control of quality, and medical have all utilized FT-NMR technologies. One of the most well-known uses of FT-NMR is the use of magnetic resonance imaging (MRI).

Disadvantages of FT-NMR:

An NMR spectrum can be obtained using the Fourier transform for NMR (FT-NMR) technique, which simultaneously excites every nucleus of a molecule that contains a certain isotope (e.g., 1 H, 13 C, etc.), using a pulse of radio waves. The following are some drawbacks of the Fourier transform in NMR:

- The Fourier Transform (FT) may not effectively represent signals with high amounts of noise since it is noise sensitive.
- Given the length of the data and the quantity of frequencies that have to be examined, it could be computationally expensive.
- Analysis of non-periodic signals that are especially speech or randomized signals, is not appropriate.

Applications of FT-NMR:

- The framework and behaviour of molecules in solution are investigated using the potent analytical approach known as Fourier transformation Nuclear Magnetic Resonance (FT-NMR). It has a wide range of applications in many disciplines, including chemistry, medicine, biology, and the study of materials.
- FT-NMR depends on the examination of the complicated time-domain output produced by the sample using the Fourier transform. Through this process, the signal is transformed into a comprehensible frequency-domain spectrum. There are numerous uses for FT-NMR, including:
- Determination of structure: Small chemical compounds, peptides from and natural and manufactured products can all have their structures determined using FT-NMR.
- FT-NMR can be utilized in the study of metabolism to locate and measure compounds in biological specimens.
- Determining the molecular makeup of proteins in solution: FT-NMR may be used to accomplish this.
- Inspection of quality: Organic compound clarity and composition can be determined using FT-NMR.
- Since it doesn't harm the sample, FT-NMR provides a non-destructive method. It is also extremely accurate and capable of detecting analytical substances at low levels of concentration. It is a useful tool for numerous uses in both research and manufacturing because to its unique characteristics.

References

1. H. Kuar, instrumental methods of chemical analysis, pragati prakashan, 4th edition, pages 421
2. Basic principles of FT NMR article from ©Gerd Gemmecker,1999.
3. Alain Louis-Joseph, Designing and building a low-cost portable FT-NMR spectrometer in 2019, A modern challenge, 2019 pages 695-711
4. Willard, Instrumental methods of analysis, CBS, 7th edition, December 2004.

Questions

1. Write a note on components of FT-NMR.
2. Add a note on advantages, disadvantages and applications of FT-NMR.

CHAPTER 11

Capillary Electrophoresis-Mass Spectroscopy (CE-MS)

Introduction

One essential micro-separation method used in studies on the environment, biotechnology, and the life sciences is high-performance capillary electrophoresis (HPCE). In comparison to traditional analytical separation techniques, it offers great separation efficiency, fast speed, and efficiency of sample size. Since demonstrating great efficiency in separation for the first time, CE has grown tremendously and is now demonstrating unmatched resolution capability for condensed-phase separations. It is especially helpful for assessing small sample sizes and intricate biological combinations. However, high detection sensitivity is also required due to CE's poor load capabilities, which has prompted initiatives to enhance CE technology.

The method has undergone a thorough evaluation, and mass spectrometry, also known as MS, is progressively being used when combined with it as recognition of its significance grows. The issues faced by analytical chemists include the need to create highly effective method of separation with precise and sensitive detectors due to the diminishing sample volumes and rising sample heterogeneity. With its great specificity and sensitivity, the mass spectrometer is a detector for quantitative separations that is both selective and widely applicable. It can provide information about unidentified substances present in mixes of samples.

Principle: High effectiveness and CE are combined together exceptional selectivity as well as high specificity detection in CE-MS. Rapid speed provided by MS. Separation based on the mass-to-charge proportion of an analyte after first being based upon the charge-to-size ratio. Dividing a sample's ionic components first by subjecting it to electricity.

Instrumentation: Components involves:

- Capillary Electrophoresis

- Interfaces
- Mass unit

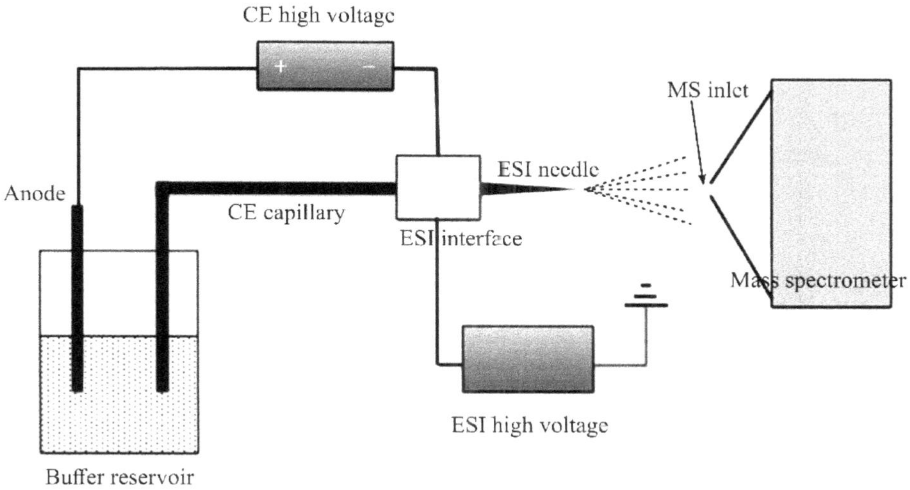

Fig.11.1 Instrumentation of CE-MS.
https://images.app.goo.gl/UmfH9tcaNjnAPewL7

- **Capillary electrophoresis:**

Using a voltage that is applied of 1000 volts per centimeter, the procedure of capillary electrophoresis is a technique for analysis that differentiates ions according to their electrophoretic movement.

Both the anode and the cathode are connected to form a capillary.

Two interactions that cause components to travel down the capillary.

1. Electrophoretic mobility
2. The flow of electrolytes or electro osmotic flow

1. **Electrophoretic mobility:** Transportation of particles that are charged in a stagnant medium caused by an electric field being generated is known as electrophoretic mobility (Map). The positively charged cathode is approached by the positive electrons.
2. **Electro osmotic flow:** An ionization of groups of silanol on fused silica results in charged sites across the inside wall of the capillary. The capillaries electrically inert surface communicates with the positive substance. The components are effectively separated by the EOF and electrophoretic movement. By definition, the zeta value at the solvent/silica interaction causes the separation buffer to move within the silica capillary. Slow EOF is brought on by very poor silanol

molecule ionization at extremely low pH levels. A rise in pH causes a boost in the number of ionized sites, which raises EOF. Maximal EOF and maximal ionization sites at extremely high pH.

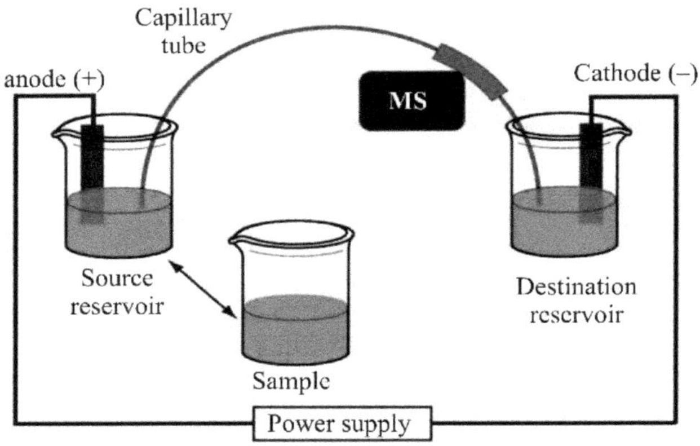

Fig.11.2 Electro osmotic flow.
Chem.libretexts.org/Courses/Northeastern_University/12: Chromatographic and Electrophoretic_Methods/12.7: Electrophoresis.

- **Interfaces:** Analytes can now be successfully transferred continuously from electrophoretic capillaries to mass spectroscopy instruments using mass spectrometry (MS) and electrophoretic ionization (CE) techniques without sacrificing separation efficiency. Because of their propensity for heat degradation, polar molecules are difficult to separate using traditional ionization methods. This is where CE shines. Over the past ten years, several new ionization techniques have been developed, such as matrix-assisted laser desorption ionization (MALDI), rapid atom bombardment (FAB), thermospray (TSP), atmospheric pressure ionization (API) techniques, and plasma resorption (PD). For MS detection in CE-MS, the ionization process must be directly coupled to liquid-phase separation methods. Reproducibility and reliability of the interface have improved recently.

  Most recently used interfaces are:

  - Electrospray ionization (ESI)
    1. Sheath flow interface
    2. Sheath less interface
    3. Liquid junction interface
  - Continuous flow fat atom bombardment
  - Matrix assisted laser desorption ionization (MALDI)

- **Electron Spray Ionization (ESI)**

Charged droplets generated at the ESI capillary tip, solvent loss and breakdown and gas-phase ion generation are the four main processes involved in ESI-MS. Ion evaporation, desolvation, and secondary reactions are all involved in the process. Since its initial demonstration in 1917, ESI has significantly transformed the analysis of amino acid sequence and molecular mass in protein biochemistry studies. Recent discoveries have revealed multiple charged species with an ESI interface, and the sheath-flow and sheathless ESI interface types have become widely accepted for CE-ESI-MS.

It is a method of evaporation. sample delivered by the capillary. A strong current will be supplied to the capillary's tip. Nebulizing gas is given with nitrogen to aid in the spraying of the analyzer sample. Heated nitrogen gas is used as the desolvation gas, which aids in vaporizing the material. There is a considerable possibility for ionization of droplets. The solvent will evaporate in the presence of heating desolvation gas, producing atomic ions.

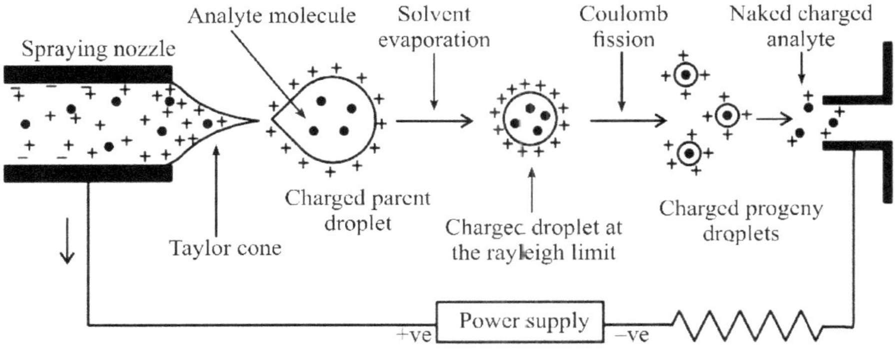

Fig.11.3 Electron spray ionization (ESI).

https://images.app.goo.gl/s9Ym5o4xbdiEMvHv7

1. **Sheath flow interface**: This is made up of two stainless steel tubes: the outer layer of liquid tube and the middle tube, referred to as the CE capillary. Between that tube and the interior of the CE capillary, the sheath fluid flows. The nebulizing airflow that enables the nebulizing process flows through the sheathing liquid pipe and the third and final outer tube, also known as the glass tube. For this kind of interface, an external concentric passageway to the CE capillaries continuously injects a sheath liquid into the nebulizer.

   At the extremities of the ESI nebulizer, the background electrolyte (BGE) and the sheath fluid are forming a junction and spraying simultaneously.

Sheen fluid: Often employed: 1:1 water-to-methanol mixture with 0.1% acetic or formic acid as the solvent. Since the outer layer of liquid is linked to the CE output electrode, the junction that forms with the background electrolyte (BGE) makes it possible to keep the magnetic field in place. Regardless of the electroosmotic flow, which causes the EOF in CE to be of an order of 20–200 nL/min, the electrospray process works most effectively at rates of flow in the μL/min range. Consequently, there is an obvious difference between the EOF and the electrospray needs. The sheath liquid provides a make-up liquid to adjust the discharge flow to the electrospray needs. High voltage is delivered to the capillary's intake side in the CE-MS coupling, and there is also an elevated voltage potentially between the spraying needle and the endplates close to the capillary where the MS entry is located.

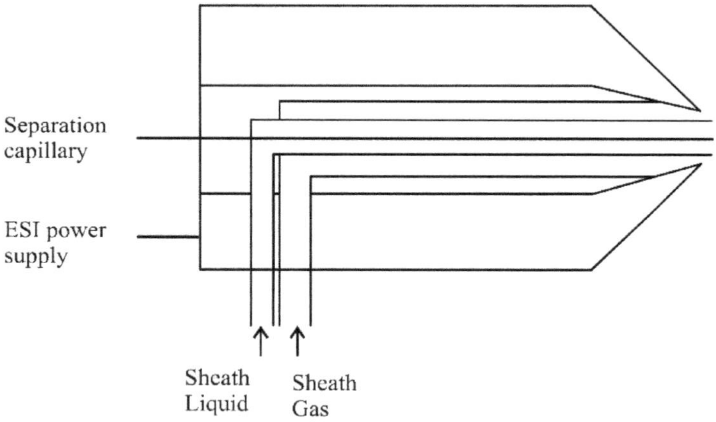

Fig.11.4. Sheath flow Interface.
https://images.app.goo.gl/VSosMi85mormJ94E7

2. **Sheath less interface:** Through a sheath-less interface system, an ESI source is directly connected to a CE capillary. Capillaries coated in conductive metal are used to create the electric collision for ESI. The equipment has minimal background information, low rate of flow, and high sensitivity since no envelope liquid is used. There are several issues with these connection designs, such as poor repeatability and low mechanical reliability.

   The newest sheath-less interface design uses a chemical etching process to create a porous ESI the point of emission. The design successfully overcomes the issues with consistency related to earlier versions and offers strong interface with mass spectrometry methods.

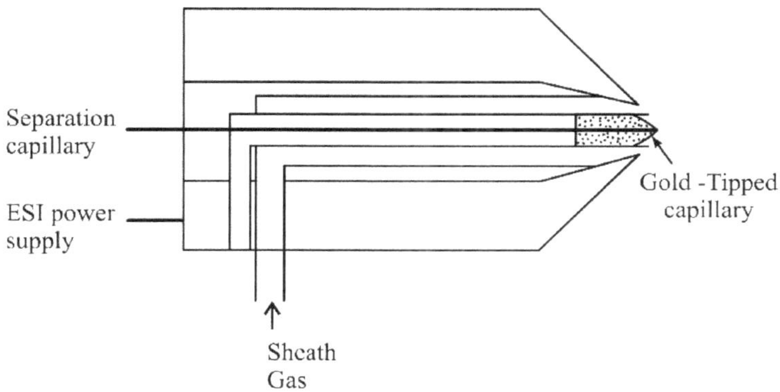

Fig.11.5 Sheath less Interface.
https://images.app.goo.gl/VScsMi85mormJ94E7

3. **Liquid junction interface:** Henion and associates created a liquid junction design that uses pneumatically assisted electrospray to couple CE to MS. The CE the capillary and ISP needle were separated by a gap of 10–25 /Lm in the stainless-steel used to construct the junction. The interface adjusted for the varying flow rates that the CE and ISP required. Synthetic drug mixtures, peptide requirements, tryptic absorbs, sulfonylurea herbicides as well sulfonated azo dyes, and drug-related substances from human urine have all been identified using this method. With separation efficiencies of up to 300,000 theoretical plates, MS detection was accomplished in both positive and negative ion modes. Additionally, gel-filled CE coupled to MS has been successfully used to separate and characterize peptides, proteins, drug-protein conjugates, pharmaceutical compounds called metabolites and natural goods, dyes for textiles, organic substances, and biological warfare agent decomposition

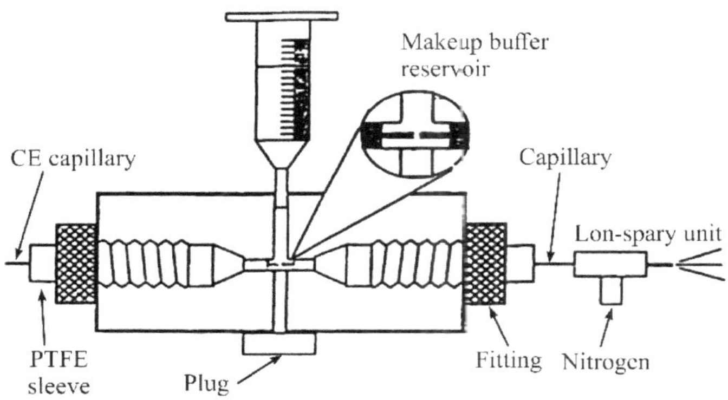

Fig.11.6 Liquid junction Interface.
https://images.app.goo.gl/VSosMi85mormJ94E7

In mass spectroscopy, using a device called an electron bombardment, a sample is transformed into quickly moving positive ions in the MS method, and the positively charged particles are sorted based on their relative weights. Electrons are thrown at organic molecules. Transformed into extremely energizing cellular ions or parent positively charged ions. Continue to fragment into smaller ions, or daughter ions. The generated ions are divided based on their mass and charge by deflection in a magnetic field.

Relative abundance (%) versus mass/charge ratio is the mass spectrum. Free radical cations are produced when a molecule loses an electron.

Advantages:

1. **High separation Efficiency:** The small tubes used in CE allow for beneficial separation efficiency. An applied electric field causes components to move at various rates, which produces exact separating.
2. **Advantages of Resolution:** The capillary tube's characteristics cause plug flow, in which the cross-sectional velocity of the tube stays constant. High resolution is achieved by reducing temperature variations and lateral diffusion. Contrary to other methods, such as the use of high-performance liquid chromatography (HPLC), CE minimizes band-broadening by maintaining a velocity that remains constant.
3. **DNA Fingerprinting:** A common advantage of CE is DNA fingerprinting. High-resolution genetic material mapping is made possible by its ability to different pieces of DNA at an accuracy of one base pair.
4. **Drug Analysis:** CE is suited for drug analysis due to its high selectivity. At particular pH levels, it can use inactive capillaries to separate substances like amines as well.
5. **Protein Characterization:** The isoelectric points that define amphoteric molecules, which are like proteins, can be used by CE to separate them. The amino acids can be recognized and described by adjusting P^H.

Disadvantages:

1. **Cost:** When compared to other methods, the starting point and machinery for CE-MS can be quite costly.
2. **Maintenance:** Over time, the capillaries utilized by CE may clog and may need to be cleaned on a regular schedule. It is imperative to maintain them neatly organized and operational.
3. **Expertise Needed:** CE-MS system operation and identifying and fixing require a greater degree of expertise. Users must comprehend the subtle differences between CE and MS.

In spite of its strength, CE-MS's empathy may be inferior to that of certain other techniques, particularly when it encounters non-UV allowing substances

Applications:

1. **Drug analysis and bioanalysis:**
    - Suitable for the analysis of drugs in a variety of matrices are drug analysis and bioanalysis.
    - When analyzing impurities.
    - Chiral examination.
    - Drug determination.
    - This includes the analysis of the ingredients in certain Chinese medicines, telandrine and fumangchinoline.
2. **Peptide and protein analysis in its intact forms:**
    - supplying disintegration data so that it can be compared with databases to find a protein or peptide that isn't known.
    - Characterization of biopharmaceuticals.
    - The top-down approach and glycoprotein analysis of proteins.
    - Evaluation of ligand-protein interactions.
    - Character development of metalloproteins.
3. **Amino acid analysis:**
    - The amino acid sequences have also been examined using CE-MS, and while the separation between the two was not entirely fixed, the MS corrected this.
    - For instance, separating and measuring amino acids found in bowel movements. a successful separation of 27 amino acids was conducted in less than 30 minutes, including the isomers are compounds of L-leucine, L-isoleucine, and L-allo iscleucine.
4. **Food omics and food analysis:**
    - CE-MS application in food quality and safety as well as other food traceability and biological function areas utilizing both traditional food analysis methods and cutting-edge food omics techniques.
5. **Biochemistry:**
    - The goal of the quickly developing genomics functional field known as "metabolomics" is to thoroughly analyze small-molecule metabolic products in biological material.

- Without requiring laborious sample dealing with, CE-ESI-MS provides a practical arrangement for achieving separation of complicated combinations of cationic, anionic, and/or zwitterionic metabolites along with their isobaric / isomeric forms.

6. **Isometrical compound segregation:**
   - Although glucose-6-phosphate and fructose-6-phosphate share the same molecular weights and formulas for chemical compounds, LC-MS cannot separate them; however, CE-MS can quantify them. Scopolamine-treated and two stereoisomers are the result of hyoscyamine separation.

7. In forensic science, CE-MS is a potent instrument that can analyze a wide range of evidence, such as explosives, narcotics, poisons, and DNA, and it may also provide important details about the identity as well as the past of the evidence.

References

1. Gerhardus de Jong, John Wiley & Sons, Capillary Electrophoresis- Mass Spectrometry (CE-MS) Principles and Applications, 16 Jun 2016.
2. Capillary Electrophoresis- Mass Spectrometry (CE-MS) Wikipedia.
3. Jasna Hradski, Martin G, Advantages and Pitfalls of Capillary Electrophoresis of Pharmaceutical Compounds and Their Enantiomers in Complex Samples: Comparison of Hydrodynamically Opened and Closed Systems, International Journal of Molecular Sciences, 18 September 2020
4. Shahab A. Shamsi, Capillary Electrophoresis Mass Spectrometry: Developments and Applications for Enantioselective Analysis, 2022 Jun 21
5. Jianyi Cai, Jack Henion, A Review Capillary electrophoresis-mass spectrometry, Analytical Toxicology, capillary electrophoresis (CE)-mass spectrometry (MS), Journal of Chromatography A, pages 667-692

Questions

1. Write about interfaces of CE-MS.
2. Add a note on applications, advantages and disadvantages of CE-MS.

CHAPTER 12

Inductively Coupled Plasma-Mass Spectrometry (ICP-MS)

Introduction

ICP-MS is an analytical method used for trace metal analysis in biological fluids. Despite some outdated methods like atomic absorption and emission, ICP-MS has gained popularity in the past decade. For almost 30 years, laboratories worldwide have used ICP-MS for trace metal analyses. While ICP and AA Plasma-optical emission systems still dominate inorganic analysis, ICP-MS is gaining ground in labs with minimal detection limits and high productivity needs.

Principle: The sample introduction system involves nebulizing liquid samples to create a fine aerosol, which is then delivered to the argon plasma. The plasma atomises and ionizes the sample, extracting ions through ion optics. The ion beam is directed into a quadrupole mass analyzer, which separates ions based on their mass-charge ratio (m/z) and measures them using a detector.

Instrumentation:

The instrumentation of ICP-MS mainly includes following parts. They are:

1. Sample introduction system
2. Torch
3. Interface
4. Ion optics
5. Mass analyzer
6. Detector.

1. Sample introduction system:

ICP-MS instruments are typically designed for liquid analysis, while electro -thermal vaporization and laser ablation can be used for solid material analysis in clinical biochemistry laboratories.

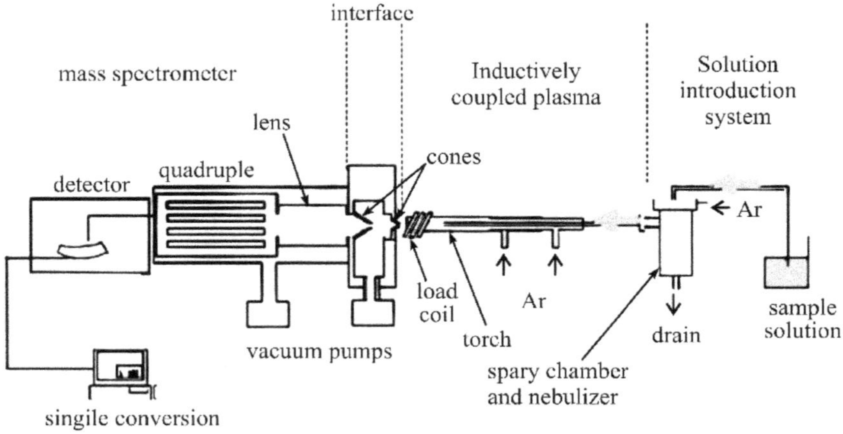

Fig.12.1 Instrumentation of ICP-MS.
https://images.app.goo.gl/QcQ7i6VjMHEbTLn39

Liquid preparation:

Liquid samples are aerosolized by a nebulizer before entering the ICP, typically using an autosampler and peristaltic pump, although self-aspirating nebulizers also available.

Nebulizer:

Nebulizers, available in various designs like pneumatic, ultrasonic, and desolvating models, are commonly used in clinical applications. Pneumatic nebulizers, such as concentric, cross-flow, Babington, and v-groove, are popular for creating aerosols using gas flow. The choice depends on the application and has its own benefits and cons.

Concentric nebulizers are ideal for low matrix samples, while cross-flow and v-groove nebulizers are durable and can handle high matrix materials. Ultrasonic nebulizers use sound energy to develop aerosols, increasing analytical sensitivity but being more costly. Desolvating nebulizers use a heated spray chamber to increase sensitivity and reduce oxide species production in plasma, which can obstruct some analyte detection.

Spray chamber:

The nebulizer creates an aerosol from the sample, which enters a spray chamber. This chamber filters out larger particles and smooths out nebulization pulses. Large droplets, over 10 m in diameter, are difficult for plasma to separate. Aerosol droplets exit the nebulizer and pass through a central tube in a two-pass spray chamber. Smaller droplets are transmitted to the plasma, while larger droplets, escaping the chamber under gravity, are drained to trash.

Cyclonic spray chambers, designed differently but functioning similarly, have a significantly ineffective sample introduction procedure compared to methods like graphite furnace atomic absorption. Only 1% to 2% of the sample makes it to the plasma, with the rest drained. Variables like the temperature of the spray chamber, typically maintained at 2°C, can significantly impact instrument response. This temperature minimizes oxide production and prevents solvent overflow of the plasma, ensuring accurate results.

2. Torch:

The ICP torch produces highly hot plasma, which is 6000°C hotter than the sun's surface, 10 times hotter than a pizza oven, and three times hotter than a welding torch. The plasma is created by flowing argon through a concentric quartz tube wrapped by an RF coil with the coil's energy from the RF generator combining with the argon.

The liquid droplets carrying the sample matrix and the elements to be identified are dried to a solid and then heated to a gas as they travel through the plasma. More energy is taken up by the atoms as they move through the plasma, and finally they release one electron to produce singly charged ions. Ions that are solely charged leave the plasma and move into the area of the interface.

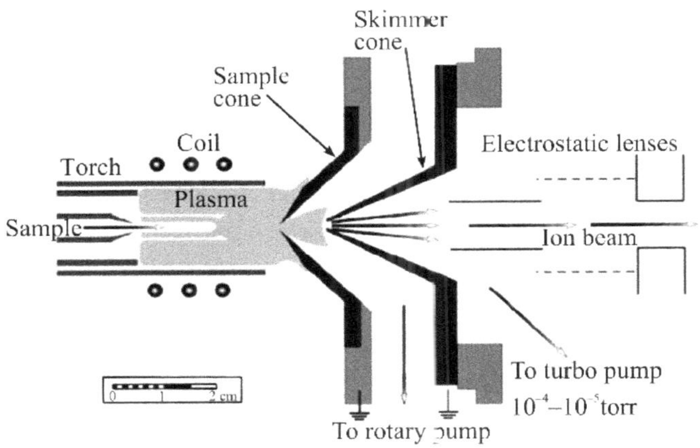

Fig12.2 Interface of ICP-MS.
https://images.app.goo.gl/EyWtXS7bvWu7Qndc6

3. Interface:

The mass spectrometer uses a vacuum chamber and plasma separated by nickel or platinum cones. The sample cone is the first in contact with the plasma, while the skimmer cone is the second. A small aperture extracts ions, photons, and neutral atoms from the plasma. A mechanical roughing pump is used to maintain an interface pressure of **150-300 Pa** between the cones.

The instrument's components, including the RF coil and interface cones, are connected by a constant flow of cooling fluid to prevent overheating. The ions approach the interface area, causing a sudden drop in pressure, resulting in a supersonic expansion, creating a free jet. The primary vacuum chamber is maintained at high vacuum, and ions are steered by electrostatic lenses.

4. Ion optics:

The term "ion optics" refers to the collection of electrostatic lenses that are housed underneath the skimmer cone. The ion optics system's function is to direct the ion beam in the direction of the mass analyzer while blocking photons and other neutral species, such non-ionized matrix components, from getting to the detector. While photons serve as the foundation for measurement in atomic emission methods like flame photometry and ICP-AES, if they are allowed to enter the detector they can cause noise and signal instability in ICP-MS. The ion optics often avoid this by placing a "photon-stop" (also known as a "shadow-stop") in the ion path or by deflecting the ion beam.

The design of ion optics and interfaces my varies with different manufacturers.

5. Mass analyzer:

The mass spectrometer is a crucial tool in ICP-MS systems, separating singly charged ions from one another. Commercial ICP-MS systems use **quadrupole, time-of-flight, and magnetic sector mass spectrometers,** with quadrupole mass spectrometers being preferred due to their cost-effectiveness and performance. To maintain stability within rods and flow through to the detector, a quadrupole must be configured with specific voltages and radio frequencies. Different ions' mass-to-charge ratios cause instability in the cell, causing them to expel. Electronics can quickly adjust the quadrupole's settings to allow ions with different ratios to flow through.

The ICP-MS uses a sequential quadrupole to scan at a speed of over 5000 atomic mass units per second, allowing one mass to pass through at a time. This allows for the rapid identification of numerous distinct elements, despite the sequential nature of the device.

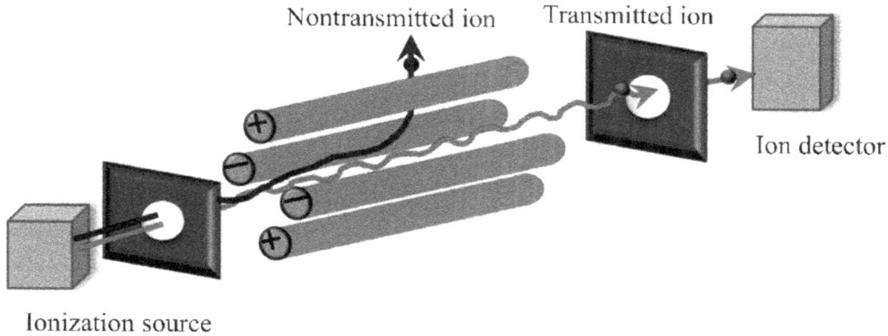

Fig.12.3 Quadrupole Mass Analyzer.
https://images.app.goo.gl/PQfLFviKz2HUebbk9

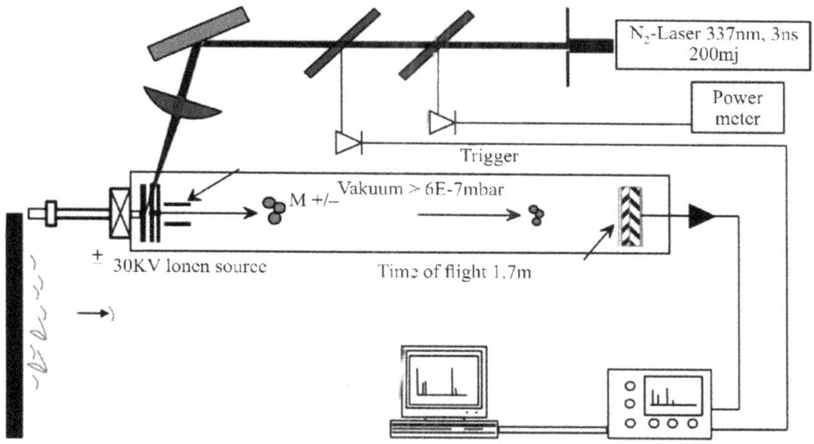

Fig.12.4 Time of Flight.
https://images.app.goo gl/MgFB6dYzaGKLhNFV7

6. Detector:

The **channeltron electron multiplier** is a commonly used ion detector in ICP-MS setups. It uses a cone-shaped tube with a high voltage opposite to the ions being detected. Ions exit the quadrupole are drawn to the cone's internal surface, releasing additional secondary electrons. As they move further into the tube, more secondary electrons are released. This process can create up to 108 electrons at the opposite end of the tube after one ion impacts.

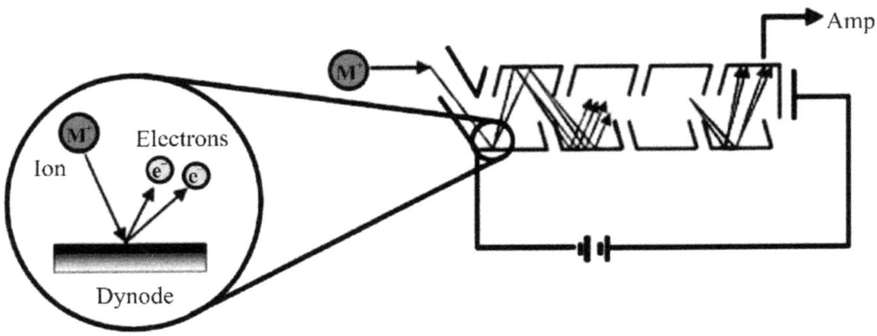

Fig.12.5 Electron Multiplier.
https://images.app.goo.gl/vorKBXGbgvxrtBUQ7

Advantages:

- High sample efficiency
- Low volume of the sample
- Convenient sample preparation
- Multi-element approach
- Large analytical range
- Minimal detection limit
- High level of interference control
- High resolution.

Disadvantages:

- Equipment and operating costs are high
- Required many high purity gases
- High degree of competence of the staff
- Interferences must be managed
- Costs associated with setting up a laboratory (air conditioning, HEPA filters, piping, dust control techniques).

Applications:

1. **Environmental monitoring:**

   ICP-MS is crucial for environmental monitoring and analysis, enabling the identification and measurement of contaminants and trace elements in air, water, soil, and sediment. It supports pollution evaluation, ecosystem investigation, and regulatory standards compliance.

- **Applications in geology and mining:**

  In geology and mining, it aids in determining ore grade, exploring resources, understanding geological processes, and assessing environmental impact of mining operations.

2. **Food and farming:**
   - ICP-MS is crucial for food safety and agriculture by analyzing food items, crops, and animal feed.
   - It helps identify pollutants like heavy metals, pesticides, and hazardous substances, and monitors nutrient content in agricultural techniques.
3. **Clinical and pharmaceutical applications:**
   - In pharmaceuticals, it tests trace elements, studies medication formulations, and detects contaminants.
   - It supports research on metal toxicity, deficiencies, biomonitoring, and clinical medication monitoring.
4. **Forensic science:**
   - ICP-MS is utilized in forensic science for elemental analysis of trace evidence, aiding in investigations and criminalistics.
5. **Material science and industrial applications:**
   - Used for monitoring and controlling elemental impurities in metals, alloys, ceramics, and electronic components, ensuring product integrity and adherence to industry standards.
6. **Health care and biomedical research:**
   - ICP-MS is utilized in health and biomedical research to analyze metal toxicity, examine disorders, and explore metal biochemistry.
   - It aids in understanding environmental exposure's impacts on human health and metal absorption, distribution, and metabolism in biological systems.
7. **Nuclear energy and radiochemistry:**
   - It is crucial for nuclear safety, radioisotope tracking, and environmental monitoring of radioactive pollutants.

References

1. Scott C Wilschefski and Matthew R Baxter, Inductively Coupled Plasma Mass Spectrometry: Introduction to Analytical Aspects, Clin Biochem Rev,2019 Aug; 40(3): 115–133
2. The 30-Minute Guide to ICP-MS, Perkin Elmer

3. Mahesh. B , Baburao .C, Bhargavi. S, Sreekanth.N and Sreenu .D, Inductively Coupled Plasma Mass Spectrometry, International journal of research in pharmacy and chemistry, 2012, 2(3), ISSN: 2231–2781
4. 2 Key Points to Know What Is ICP-MS: Working Principle and Applications, Drawell analytical chemistry

Questions

1. Brief about the detector used in the ICP-MS.
2. Explain the principle involved in ICP-MS.
3. Discuss the instrumentation of ICP-MS.
4. Mention advantages and disadvantages of ICP-MS.
5. Enlist the types of nebulizers used in the ICP-MS Instrumentation.

CHAPTER 13

Inductively Coupled Plasma-Atomic Emission Spectroscopy (ICP-AES)

Introduction

The atomic emission spectrometry detector and the inductively coupled plasma source are the two fundamental components of an ICP-AES system. Atomic emission spectroscopy using inductively coupled plasma, commonly known as ICP-AES or ICP-OES (Inductively coupled Plasma – Optical Emission Spectroscopy), uses an ICP (inductively coupled plasma) to excite atoms or ions that emit electromagnetic radiation with a wavelength unique to a certain element. The strength of this emission can be used to identify the element's concentration in the sample.

Principle: In inductively coupled plasma-optical emission spectrometry, a sample is transported as a liquid stream into an instrument, converted into an aerosol through nebulization, and then transported to the plasma for desolvation, vaporization, atomization, and excited/ionization. The excited atoms and ions emit characteristic radiation, which is collected by a device that sorts it by wavelength. The radiation is detected and converted into electronic signals, providing concentration information for the analyst.

Instrumentation:

The main components of ICP-AES instrumentation is:

1. Nebulizer
2. Pumps
3. Spray chamber
4. Drains
5. Radio frequency generator
6. Torch
7. Transfer optics
8. Wavelength dispersive devices
9. Detectors
10. Computers and processor

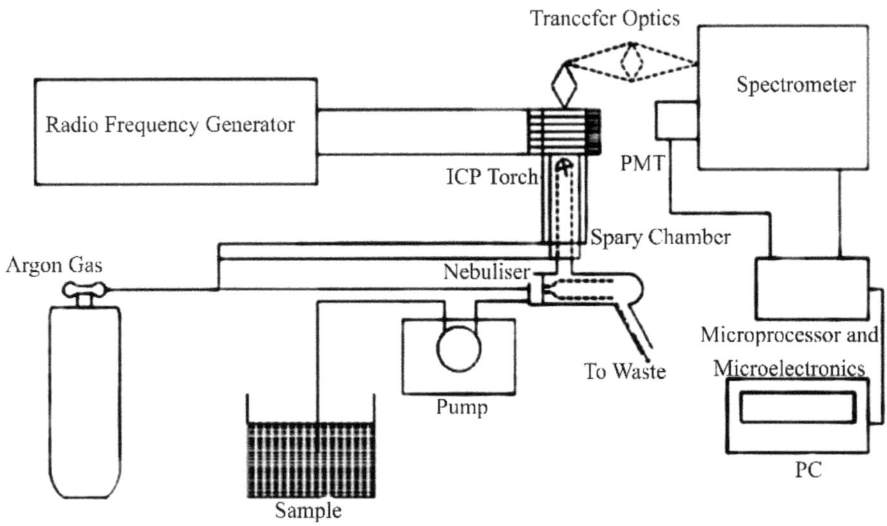

Fig. 13.1 Instrumentation of ICP-AES.
https://images.app.goo.gl/XBs9HohS8y7L9jJ58

1. Nebulizer:

Nebulizers convert liquids into aerosols for plasma transport, crucial in ICP-OES. The ideal sample introduction mechanism ensures high reproducible of desolvation, evaporation, atomize, ionization, and excitation. The nebulizer's ability to produce small droplets is crucial.

Mostly used nebulizers are:

I. Concentric nebulizer
II. Micro-concentric nebulizer
III. Cross flow nebulizer
IV. Babington nebulizer

I. Concentric nebulizer: This nebulizer uses a capillary tube to deliver a solution to a low-pressure area, breaking it into an aerosol. The orifices are smaller than those in flame spectrometers due to lower sample aerosol carrier flow. Concentric pneumatic nebulizers offer good sensitivity and stability, but solutions with as low as 0.1% dissolved particles may cause clogging issues. Design improvements have increased their tolerance to dissolved solids.

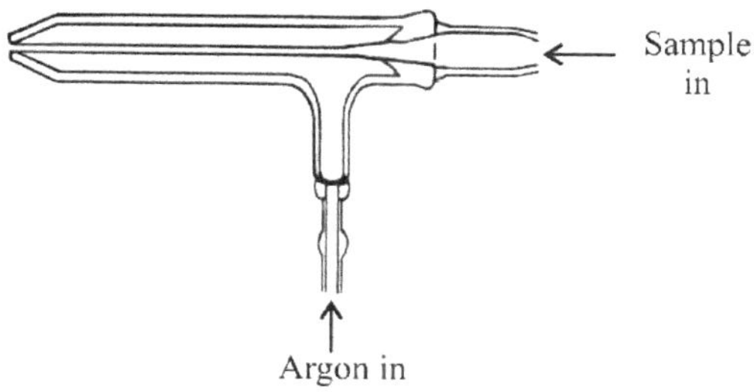

Fig.13.2 Concentric Nebulizer.
https://images.app.goo.gl/4ik8uDNLTo2GC7aw9

II. Micro-concentric nebulizer: The nebulizer's low sample uptake and quick washout durations make it a unique device for multi-element analysis, extending the required sample volumes and reducing nebulization times. Its limited sample capacity and low uptake rates make it effective.

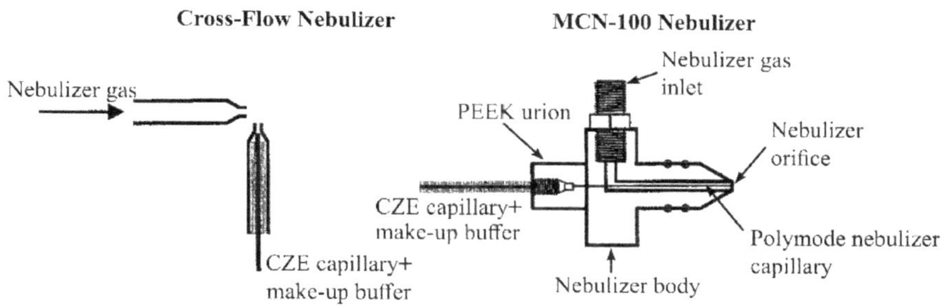

Fig.13.3 Cross flow and Micro-concentric Nebulizers.
https://images.app.goo.gl/NwcZRH1EPrWsRfTy5

III. Cross flow nebulizer: Cross-flow nebulizer activity is similar to perfume atomizers, where a capillary tube's tip is perpendicular to a high-speed argon gas stream. This gas creates a low-pressure area, either drawing the solution or using a pump, causing liquid fragmentation into an aerosol.

Concentric nebulizers produce smaller droplets for ICP analysis than cross-flow nebulizers due to larger diameter capillaries and greater separation between liquid and gas injectors. Cross-flow nebulizers are durable and corrosion-resistant, making them a better choice.

IV. Babington nebulizer: This nebulizer uses a smooth surface with a tiny hole to nebulize viscous liquids, ripping them into tiny drops using fast-moving argon gas.

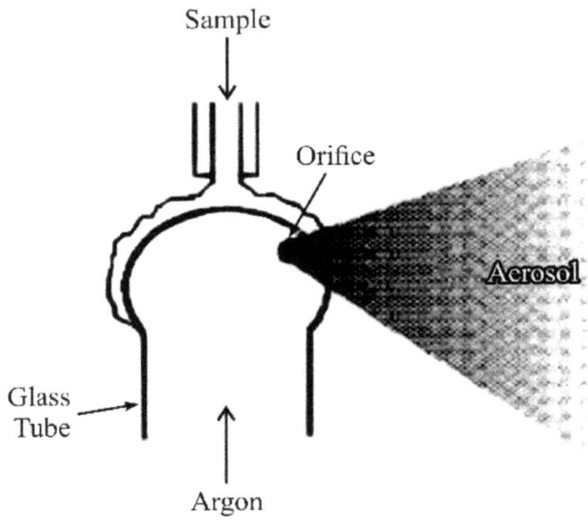

Fig.13.4 Babington Nebulizer.
https://images.app.goo.gl/WaVCv8VkyVhowa3z8

2. **Pumps:** Babington types, like V-groove and ultrasonic, and some nebulizers require solution conveyance. Cross-flow and concentric nebulizers can naturally aspirate solution, but a pumped flow is also effective.

   Peristaltic pumps are the preferred choice for ICP-OES applications due to their peristalsis mechanism, which uses rollers to force sample solution down tubing. This ensures that only the tubing contacts the pump, eliminating the risk of solution contamination with other pumps.

   Peristaltic pump tubing must be compatible with the sample it's pumping through, with most types being compatible with weakly acidified aqueous media. However, specific tubing is needed for acidic solutions or organic solvents. Peristaltic pump tubing requires regular repair in an ICP system.

3. **Spray chamber:** The nebulizer produces sample aerosol, which is then injected into plasma using a spray chamber between the nebulizer and torch. The chamber removes large droplets and eliminates pulses from solution pumping during nebulization, ensuring only tiny droplets are suitable for plasma injection.

   ICP spray chambers allow droplets with diameters of 10 µ to pass through to plasma, forming 1%-5% of sample introduction to a standard nebulizer, with 95-99% residual material disposed of in a waste container.

4. **Drains:** The ICP instrument's performance may be affected by the drain system, which transports extra samples from the spray chamber to a waste container, creating backpressure needed to drive the nebulizer gas through the torch injector tube.

5. **Radio frequency generator:** The plasma discharge is created and maintained by a radio frequency (RF) generator, which delivers power to the plasma gas through a load coil. The coil, typically copper tubing, is cooled by water or gas and functions as an antenna. Most RF generators for ICP-OES operate between 27 and 56 MHz.
6. **Torch:** The argon flow and aerosol injection in torches are carried out through three concentric tubes, with narrow spaces between them for high velocity escape. The gas spirals tangentially around the outside chamber, known as the "outer" gas flow, to keep the quartz walls of the torch cold. The typical outside gas flow for argon ICPS is 7-15 liters per minute.

   Gas is sent under the plasma toroid through the chamber, simplifying the sample aerosol's entrance and diverting plasma discharge from the injector and intermediate tubes. This flow, originally known as the auxiliary flow, is approximately 1.0 L/min when the torch is operating normally.

   The sample aerosol is introduced into the plasma via a central tube or injector, which can even penetrate the plasma with a 1 L/min argon nebulization.

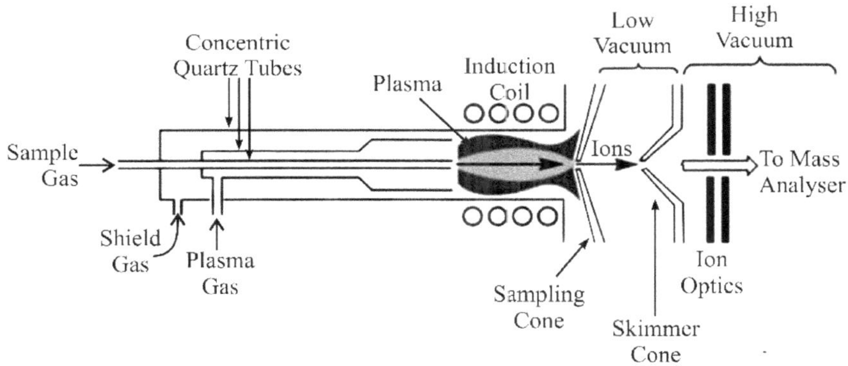

Fig.13.5 Torch used in ICP-AES.
https://images.app.goo.gl/oAAgJTzMrQGCFyWP8

7. **Transfer optics:** For the spectrometric measurement, a sample of the emission radiation from the plasma's normal analytical zone (NAZ) is taken. In recent years, the analytical zone working in a vertical orientation was seen from the side of the plasma. A radial or side-on viewing of the plasma is the term used to describe this traditional method of ICP spectroscopy. The zone is viewed from the end of the plasma after it has been rotated to a horizontal position. This arrangement of the ICP is now referred to as an axial or end-on viewpoint.

Dual vision instruments, which integrate radial and axial viewing, have recently been introduced. Typically, a focusing optic like a convex lens or a concave mirror collects the radiation. The image of the plasma is then focused by this optic onto the entry slit of the spectrometer or wavelength dispersing device.

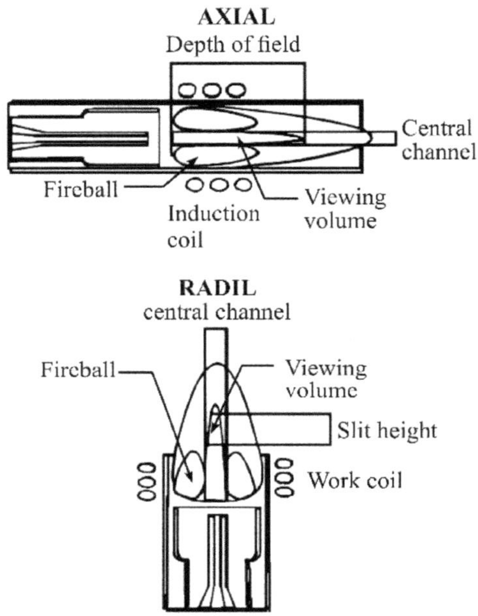

Fig.13.6 Axial and Radial view point.
https://images.app.goo.gl/drAJkAnjkHn2Bgkr5

8. **Wavelength dispersive devices:** ICP-OES analyses are typically conducted using dispersive devices with **diffraction gratings**, which are mirrors with closely spaced lines. These gratings have a line density ranging from 600 to 4200 lines per millimeter and diffracted light at an angle influenced by the wavelength and line density. The angle of diffraction is typically higher for longer wavelengths and higher line density.

   A spectrometer uses a grating to separate polychromatic light into monochromatic radiation. It focuses light into a precise beam and disperses it according to wavelength. The scattered light is concentrated onto a circle or exit plane, allowing some wavelengths to reach the detector while obstructing others. The spectrometer's job is to perform this process according to wavelength, ensuring accurate and reliable results.

The majority of monochromatic radiation diffracted from the grating is composed of wavelengths that correspond to the light emitted by a specific elemental or chemical species in the ICP.

9. **Detectors:** The photomultiplier tube (PMT), also known as the detector, is the most commonly used detector for ICP-OES, used to measure the intensity of the emission line after the correct emission line is separated by the spectrometer.

   The photocathode in a Photomolecular Transporter (PMT) releases electrons when exposed to light. These are directed towards a dynode, which ejects two to five secondary electrons for every primary electron. This creates a multiplicative effect, with PMTs having 9 to 16 dynode phases. The last phase is the capture of secondary electrons.

   A nine-dynode PMT can produce up to 106 secondary electrons from a single photon, determining its relative intensity using electrical current. This technology offers advantages over other detection methods, including the ability to amplify low emission levels and span nine orders of magnitude in light intensity.

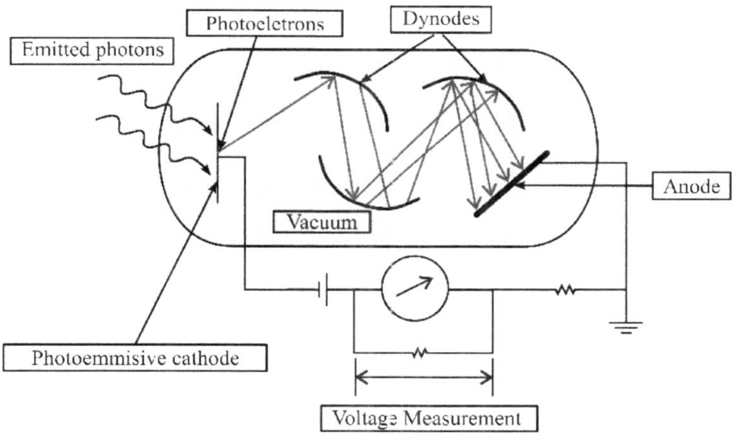

Fig. 13.7 Photomultiplier Tube.
https://images.app.goo.gl/JmfgTiMFUHR7yu2L6

Advanced array detector:

Three advanced solid-state detectors, the photodiode array (PDA), charge-injection device (CID), and charge-coupled device (CCD), have been developed for spectroscopic applications. These devices, part of the charge transfer devices (CTD) class, are based on the light-sensitive properties of solid-state silicon. They offer high sensitivity and resolution, making them a valuable tool in various applications.

Advantages:

- Major, minor, and trace element determination in a wide range of sample matrices is considered to be a reliable analytical task using ICP-OES, which is a strong and adaptable analytical instrument.
- High selectivity and sensitivity
- A wide dynamic range
- Minimal detection limits, multi-element detection.
- Very minimal amounts of matrix interferences are all features of the ICP-OES technology.

Disadvantages:

- Inadequate precision, sample drift, unfavorable detection limits, and imprecise identification are typical issues with ICP-OES.

Applications:

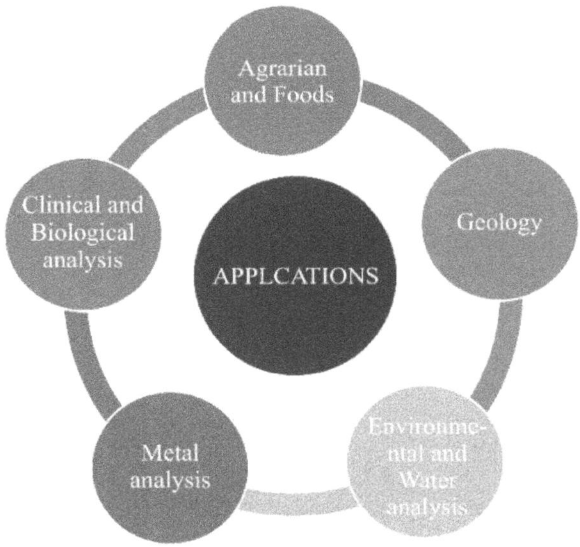
Agrarian and Foods
Geology
Environme-ntal and Water analysis
Metal analysis
Clinical and Biological analysis
APPLCATIONS

1. **Agrarian and foods:** A wide range of agricultural and culinary items have been analyzed using the ICP-OES technology. Samples can be in the form of soil, fertilizer, plant material, food, feed, animal tissues, or bodily fluids. It is necessary to determine these materials to identify their amounts of harmful components as well as important nutrients which can be analyzed by ICP-OES.

2. **Clinical and biological analysis:** ICP-OES has developed into a key instrument for biological and clinical applications as more knowledge about the functions and behaviors of trace elements in biological systems is revealed by study. Essential, toxic, and therapeutic trace element determinations by ICP-OES are critical in clinical and forensic lab settings as well as medical research labs.
3. **Geology**: ICP-OES is used in geology to analyze the major, minor, and trace compositions of diverse rocks, soils, sediments, and related materials. ICP-OES is mostly used in this industry for exploration purposes. The method is also employed in applications including ocean geochemistry and tracing the origins of rock formations.
4. **Environmental and water analysis:** Environmental ICP-OES applications include a number of water quality analyses mandated by the US Environmental Protection Agency, the determination of Fe, Cd, Cu, Mo, Ni, V, and Zn in seawater, the determination of phosphorus in municipal waste water, the determination of heavy metals in inner-city dust samples, and the analysis of trace metals in coal fly ash.
5. **Metal analysis:** ICP-OES for metals is frequently used to identify the main, minor, and trace elemental components of metals and related materials. The method is employed in the development lab setting as well as for the examination of raw materials, production control, and quality control of finished goods.

References

1. Mindy.L, ICP-OES-ICP Chemistry, ICP Analysis, strength and limitations, Technology networks, March 17, 2021
2. Maria Luisa F. Sanchez, Atomic Emission Spectrometry Inductively Coupled Plasma, Encyclopedia of Analytical Science (Third Edition), 2019.
3. Charles B. Boss and Kenneth J. Freden, Concepts, Instrumentation and Techniques in Inductively Coupled Plasma Optical Emission Spectrometry, Third edition, Perkin Elmer, inc.

Questions

1. What are the nebulizers that are used in this instrumentation?
2. List the applications of ICP-AES.
3. Enumerate the detector used in ICP-AES.
4. What is meant the side-on view and end-on view plasma?
5. Write the principle involved in ICP-AES.

CHAPTER 14

Liquid Chromatography-Tandem Mass Spectroscopy (LC-MS/MS)

Introduction

The clinical chemistry standardized metabolite methods for detection depend on indirect properties such as reactivity to chemicals or light transmission. Because mass spectrometric technologies have greater accuracy and applicability than traditional methods like the method of photometry or ligand-binding assays, it is more appealing for assessing compounds or biomarkers in diagnosing processes. Mass spectrometric technology uses fragmentation sequences and molecular weight to measure substances. After being developed over forty years ago, GC-MS is still only used in specialist settings such as toxicology labs, hospitals, and reference labs. With a daily average amount of samples of less than 50, GC-MS instrument managing along with upkeep are labour-intensive and time-consuming.

Substantial advances in technology in the past ten years have made it possible to use the liquid chromatography to organic components such as peptides, amino acids, carbohydrates, DNA, and medicines. The capacities of MS detectors have grown with the introduction of new ion-analyses technology as ion-trap MS, tandem MS, and time of flight MS. The fundamentals of mass spectrometric recognition, current advancements, and application domains in the fields of drug discovery, metabolic processes, toxicity investigations, biogenic amine measurement, doping management, and pharmacokinetics research.

Principle: Liquid chromatography-tandem mass spectroscopy is referred to as MS/MS. It is a type of analytical approach that brings together mass spectrometry's (MS) mass analysis skills with fluid chromatography's (LC) separation by matter characteristics.

Based on how the sample's constituents interact with a stationary component and a mobile phase, LC divides it separate from one another. Following the separation process, the constituents are added to the MS, where their mass-to-charge ratios allow to facilitate their detection after ionization.

A second mass spectrometer (MS) further fragments and analyzes the ions generated by the primary MS in a method known as tandem mass spectrometry (MS/MS). This offers some additional information regarding the composition and characteristics of the analytical substances. Many industries, including the field of biotechnology pharmaceuticals, monitoring the environment, food security, and medical diagnostics, depend heavily on LC MS/MS. With great sensitivity and effectiveness, it is able to identify and measure traces of analytical substances in complicated composites.

Instrumentation:

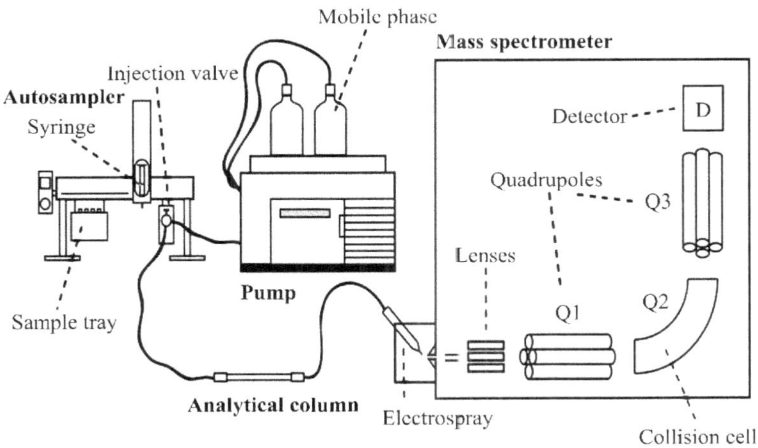

Fig.14.1 Instrumentation of LC-MS/MS.
www.researchgate.net/figure/Schematic-overview-of-a-LC-MS-MS-system-with-a-triple-quadrupole-mass-analyzer_fig7_328980854

- **Components of LC-MS/MS**
  1. LC unit
  2. Interfaces
  3. Ionization sources
  4. Mass analyzers
  5. Detectors

1. **LC unit**

   Reservoir: Inert to different aquatic and non-aqueous mobile phases; • Glass or steel made from stainless steel containers that may carry as much as one Litre of moving phase (pure solvents made from organic matter or water-based solutions of salts or buffers). Particulates is removed from the mobile phase by filtering it, and it is also degassed by vacuum, sonication, and helium sparging. Avoid using stainless steel while working with liquids that contain halide ions.

   Pumps: They deliver mobile phase with high pressure. They contain inert solvents. Three major types of pumps are used.

1. **Reciprocating pump:** Inverse flow rates of 1–15 cm^3 per minute can be produced by a reciprocating pump against column backpressures of up to 7250 psi. The pump head, which includes a piston and a solvent chamber with two check valves and a capacity as small as 0.01 cm^3, is the heart of the device. Valve one opens as the main piston exits the chamber, allow the mobile phase to enter the pump head, while valve two closes, stopping liquid from flowing out of the column. Valves one and two close as the piston makes its return stroke into the chamber and open as mobile phase is injected into the column. This procedure is repeated frequently enough to create the desired flow throughout the column.

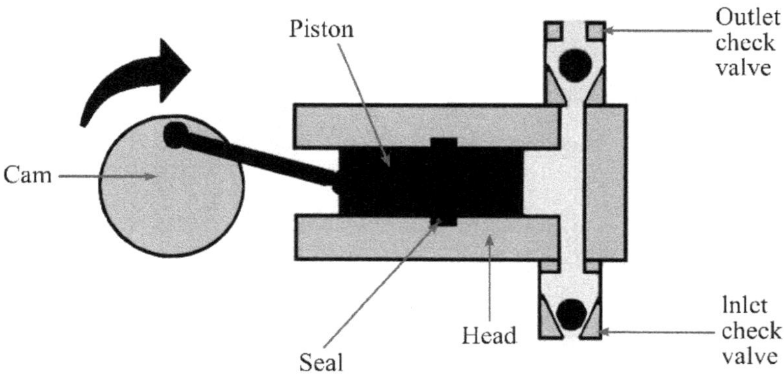

Fig.14.2 Reciprocating pump.
www.instructables.com/Simple-reciprocating-pump/

2. **Syringe pump:** These pipes work on the idea of a piston being mechanically moved at a steady pace to displace the solvent in a chamber with a 500 cm^3 volume. These pumps produce a pulse-free flow at high pressures (200–475atm).

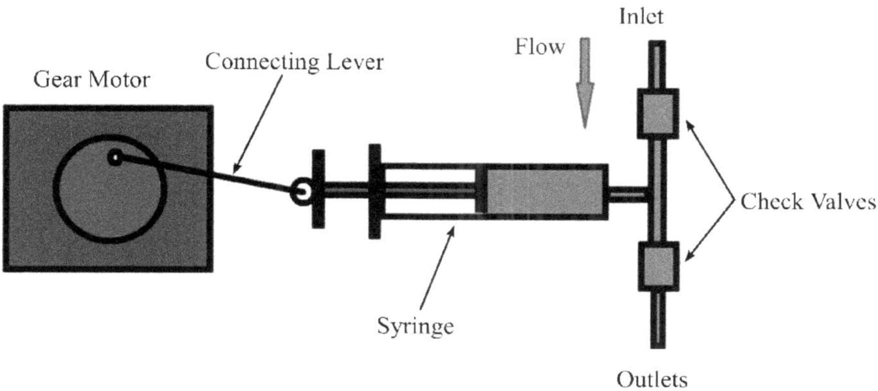

Fig.14.3 Syringe pump.
https://images.app.goo.gl/1FJRq7TWH5mJL8Xq6

3. **Constant pressure pumps:** Also called as gas displacement pump. These pumps offer non pulsating flow. These pumps have low solvent capacity.

   Gradient controller:

   A pure solvent or a combination of solvents is used to prepare the mobile phase in an isocratic separation. i.e., the same polarity or eluting power of solvent is employed. However, the solvent's polarity is gradually raised in the gradient elution approach, necessitating a change in the solvent's composition. Therefore, when two or more solvent pumps are employed for such separations, a gradient controller is needed.

4. **Injectors:** The chromatographic system's sample volume is introduced using an injector. Typically, a sample volume between 1 and 100 Liters can be injected. The injector loop allows for an increase in injection volume of up to 2 ml. There are a number of injector devices that can be used to manually or automatically inject the sample, including:
   (a) **Septum injectors:** Also called syringe injection, which are used to inject the sample through a rubber septum or self -sealing elastomer septum. Since the septum must resist high pressures, this type of injector cannot be used frequently.
   (b) **Stop Flow Injector:** In this design, the sample is injected through a valve after the mobile phase flow has been temporarily stopped.

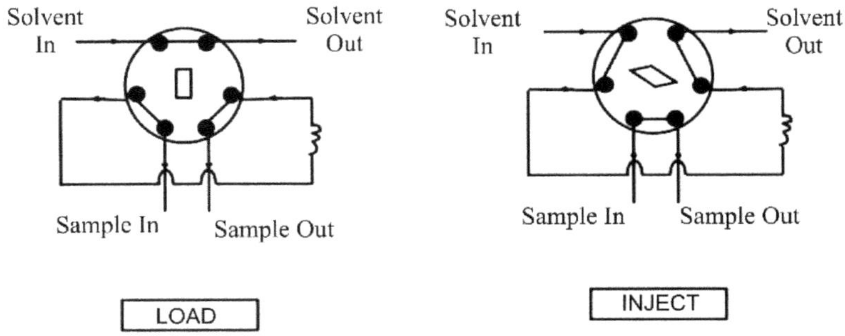

Fig.14.4 Stop Flow Injector.
www.brainkart.com/article/High-Performance-Liquid-Chromatography-%28HPLC%29--Sample-Introduction_29768/

Column: The precolumn in banded phase chromatography (LC) is coated with a high percentage of stationary phase liquid to prevent stripping of solid phase (SP) by the mobile phase. It traps particulate matter in the mobile phase, extending the life of the main analytical column. SP is permanently bonded to the support material, preventing stripping. The analytical column, the heart of the LC, is constructed from stainless steel tubes with a diameter of 2-4.6 mm and a length of 5-25 cm. It is filled with 5-10 micron-sized particles, and can be made from alumina, diatomaceous earth, or activated charcoal. The column's surface contains silanol groups.

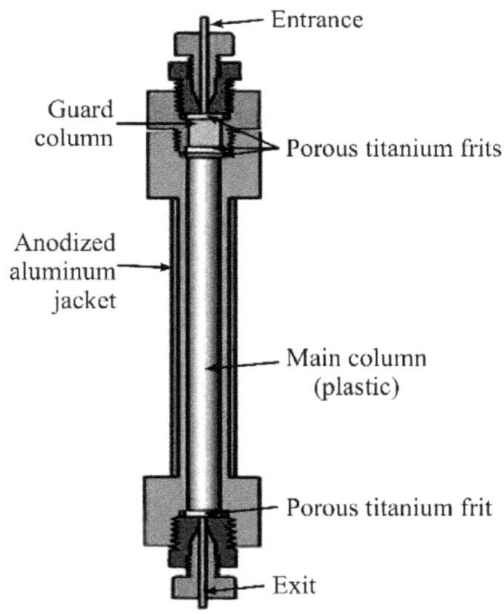

Fig.14.5 Column.
https://images.app.goo.gl/mrmKosTLV2q1cRAh8

2. **Interfaces:** A combination of liquid components, often including acetonitrile, methanol, and water, are separated using liquid chromatography. The mass spectrometer's ion source receives this liquid that contains a complex variety of components. The ion source is at a high vacuum, therefore different types of interfaces are used.

ESI (Electron Spray Ionization)

The liquid chromatography (LC) eluent flows through a metal capillary that is located inside the probe during electrospray ionization (ESI). As the LC flow exits the electrospray capillary, it nebulizes into a spray, which then condenses into droplets. By creating a significant (2–5 kV) potential difference among the electrospray capillary and counter electrode, a charge is imparted onto the droplets. By using a hot drying gas to evaporate the mobile phase, the droplet size is reduced. The charge on the surface density of the smaller droplets is increased by this desolvation. Droplet fission is caused by electric repulsion brought on by the charge density. Coulombic fission occurs when this value far exceeds the droplet's surface tension. Gas-phase ions are created as the droplet "explodes" and are normally sampled through some type of opening. Coulombic fission occurs when this exceeds the droplet's tension at the surface. The generation of protonated or deprotonated molecules with minimum fragmentation, which is optimal for the selection of precursor ions and for maximizing sensitivity, is the main benefit of using ESI for quantitative LC-MS.

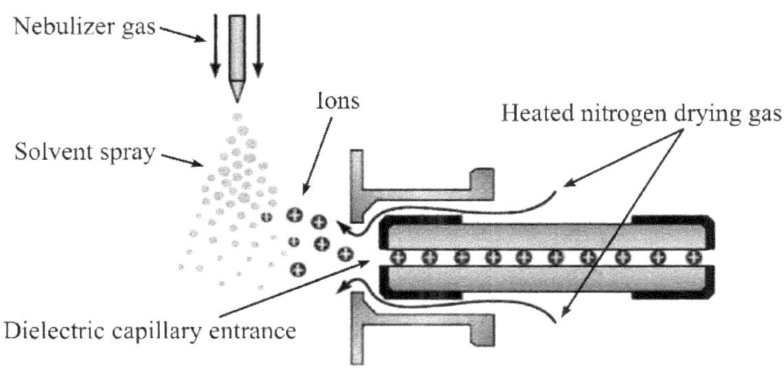

Fig.14.6 ESI (Electron Spray Ionization).
www.researchgate.net/figure/Schematic-diagram-showing-how-electrospray-ionization-works-B1_fig3_266233961

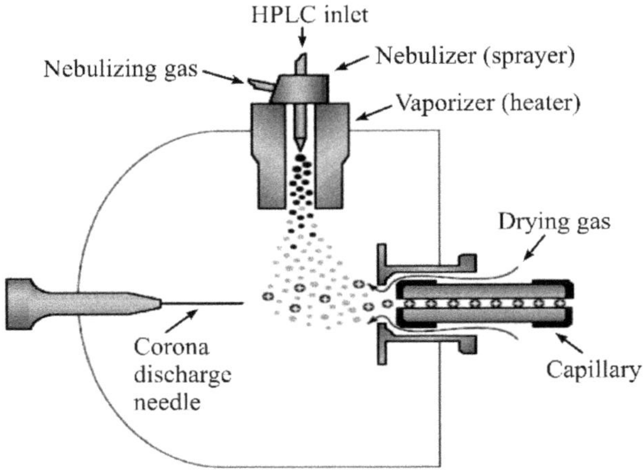

Fig.14.7 Atmospheric pressure chemical ionization.
https://analyticalsciencejournals.onlinelibrary.wiley.com/doi/abs/10.1002/mas.10060

APCI stands for atmospheric pressure chemical ionization. In APCI, the LC eluent is sprayed at atmospheric pressure over a heated (usually 250°C–400°C) vaporizer. The liquid is vaporized by the heat. Electrons released from a corona needle ionize and produce gas-phase solvent molecules. Chemical ionization is the process by which the solvent ions impart charge to the analyte molecules. A capillary sample opening allows the analyte ions to enter the mass analyser. A large variety of polar and nonpolar compounds can be used with APCI. Usually employed for molecules less than 1,500 u, it rarely leads to repeated charging. This makes APCI less suitable than electrospray for the investigation of large macromolecules that can be thermally unstable, in addition to the fact that it involves elevated temperatures.

4. Combining Liquid Chromatography with Tandem Mass Spectrometry (LC-MS/MS) OR Mass Analyzers

Tandem mass spectrometers used for sample analysis are frequently employed. These include triple quadrupole mass spectroscopy instruments (QQQ or TQMS) and the quadrupole time-of-flight (QTOF). The two quadrupole meters mass analyzers (Q1 and Q3) that make up TQMS are divided by an impact cell. To identify the precursor that is the basis of a particular product ion, Q1 and Q3 scan throughout a mass range. Q3 then monitors the precursor. Q1 simply sends the pre-specified precursor onto the collision cell; Q3, on the other hand, searches a mass range to find fragments that were obtained experimentally. By identifying all precursors which give shape to the products by the loss of exactly the same species of neutrality from all precursors that neutral loss (NL) scans through Q1 and Q3.

Because of its specificity and sensitivity, selected reactivity monitoring (SRM), which tracks particular m/z values for precursor and daughter ions, is favoured for chemical identification. Numerous precursor-to-product transformations of the same or distinct analytical substances can be monitored with a TQMS.

Triple Quadrupole Mass Analyzer:

Designers connect three quadrupoles in series, the first and third of which are mass filters and each of which functions as a single quadrupole in a triple quad system. The samples are broken up by the centre quadrupole using a collision gas, allowing for quantification of components or structural examination of samples.

SRM involves two steps of mass selection: selecting the mass of the intact targeted analyte (precursor ion) in the first quadrupole (Q1) and choosing a desired fragment (product ion) in the third quadrupole (Q3) following fragmentation of the Q1 mass-selected precursor ion by collision-induced dissociation in the second quadrupole (Q2). The desired fragment is then delivered to the detector, which records quantitative measurements based on the intensity profile of each transition. This process achieves high selectivity against co-cluting interferences, ensuring accurate measurements of the specific pair of precursor and product ions.

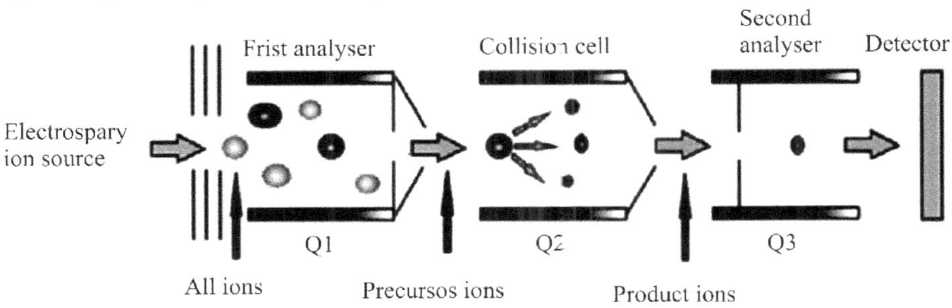

Fig.14.8 Triple quadrupole.
https://images.app.goo.gl/f4uuNawyB8jGD8EQ8

Quadrupole –TOF:

The Q-TOF-MS is a hybrid device that combines quadrupole technology with a time-of-flight mass analyzer. It is similar to a triple-quadrupole mass spectrometer, with the first quadrupole (Q1) serving as a mass filter and the second quadrupole (Q2) acting as a collision cell. The Q1 can be used in radio frequency (RF) alone mode to broadcast all icns, while the Q2 can operate in

RF-only mode without ion fragmentation. The device is similar to a triple-quadrupole mass spectrometer.

Ions exit the quadrupole and enter the time-of-flight analyzer's ion modulator section, where they are accelerated by an electric field. They reach the flight tube, where mass separation occurs. Ions with lower mass travel farther and faster. Modern time-of-flight analyzers use a reflectron device to adjust for spatial spread and kinetic energy dispersion of ions with the same m/z but different velocities.

The Q-TOF-MS detector uses reflectron adjustment to allow ions with the same m/z to enter simultaneously, enhancing mass resolution. It uses quadrupole technology and a time-of-flight analyzer to perform two types of scans for data collection. In the first mode, unfragmented precursor ions are accurately mass scanned using the first and second quadrupoles in RF-only mode. A single mass or range of masses can be chosen for transmission to the TOF analyzer using the Q1. In the second mode, ions are sent into the collision cell (Q2) for CID.

The TOF analyzer accurately quantifies the mass of product and unbroken precursor ions, while the Q-TOF-MS can simultaneously gather information on both ions by switching between modes. A time-to-digital converter is used to convert ion flight time into a mass signal.

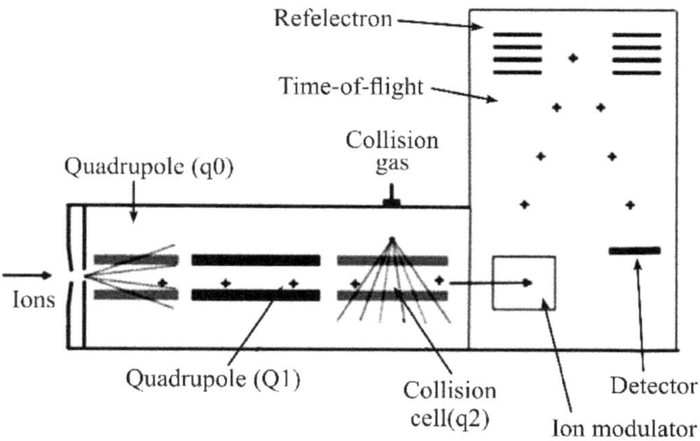

Fig.14.9 Quadrupole -TOF.
https://images.app.goo.gl/WqLJEiGJDLtJVaE57

5. Detectors:

Majorly used detectors are

1. Photo multiplier tube
2. Channel electron multiplier

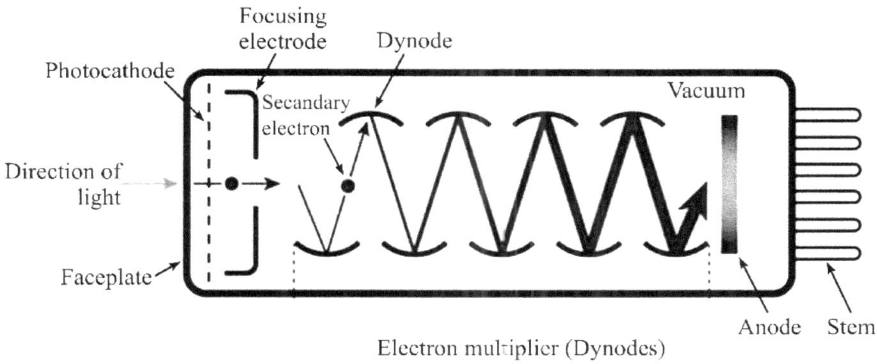

Fig.14.10 Photomultiplier tube.
www.matsusada.com/application/ps/photomultiplier_tubes/

Because metals absorb light energy, they release electrons that can be detected by PMT (photoelectric) detectors, which rely on this phenomenon. When a photon hits the first dynode, electrons are released into a higher-voltage chain. As a result, an electron cascades down the pathway until it reaches the anode, where it produces the measurable electric charge. PMT detectors allow the detection of particular photons even in low-light conditions through doubling the current generated by light that hits them by as many as 100 million times.

When light strikes a photoelectric surface, a photomultiplier tube exploits the external photoelectric response to discharge photoelectrons. Secondary electrons are released from dynodes when primary electrons release from a photoelectric surface; these electrons finally arrive at the anode's surface. To speed up the electrons and increase the secondary emissions coefficients, a high power (-HV) is supplied. Light intensity can be changed by adjusting the multiplication factor, which is accomplished by regulating the high voltage. excellent-end equipment uses photomultiplier tubes because of their excellent sensitivity and adaptability.

Advantages:

- Because of its sensitivity and selectivity, it is able to gauge and identify very low metabolite levels even in an amount of chemicals that interfere with detection.
- Because of its adaptability and broad nature, it can be used to a variety of analytes, including additives to food, medicines, biological molecules, organic compounds, pesticides, and more.
- Because of its accuracy and precision, it can produce results that are dependable, repeatable, and error-free.

- Because of its speed and efficiency, it requires little sample preparation and could separate and examine several analytes in only one analysis.

Disadvantages:

- It needs solvents and volatility buffers that work with the mass spectrometry. This restricts the selection of portable phases and may have an impact on LC's separation effectiveness.
- Molecules with poor ionization performance or those that cannot be ionizing might escape its detection. This could decrease the method's responsiveness and precision.
- If two structurally distinct isomers share the same weight and breakage patterns, it could fail to be possible to distinguish both apart. Incorrect results or inaccurate results in identification may result from it.
- It is a costly method with significant initial and recurring costs. Additionally, skilled workers are required to manage and troubleshoot the device.
- It might experience matrix implications, like ion amplification or restriction, which could have an impact on the precision performance.
- For non-volatile, polar in nature or electrically labile substances that are challenging to evaporate or fragment, it might not be the best option. Due to its manually performed nature, insufficient automated processes, low specimen efficiency, high beginning cost, technical skill, restricted standardized procedures, and absence of commercially available requirements, LC-MS/MS use for clinical diagnostics is plagued with difficulties. Most tests are generated in laboratories and need an extensive expenditure of time, cash, and expertise in technology. Manual procedures take a lot of time when it comes to analysing and presenting data. Clinical diagnostics built around proteomics were originally available at colleges and universities and a reference lab.

Applications:

- **Clinical application:**

Mass spectrometry (LC-MS/MS) has evolved from its initial use in newborn screening and diagnosing organic metabolic disorders to its current use in paediatric laboratories for newborn screening programs. Its versatility, sensitivity, and specificity make it a leading technology in paediatric laboratories for newborn screening programs. LC-MS/MS is also used in therapeutic drug monitoring (TDM) for quantitative measurement of medications, such as immunosuppressant drugs like cyclosporine A, tacrolimus, sirolimus, everolimus, and mycophenolic acid. LC-MS/MS allows for multiple analytes in one analytical run, saving time and money. It is also cost-effective for measuring anti-neoplastic agents like busulfan, which is used to calculate drug clearance and provide an estimated dose for bone marrow ablation prior to hematopoietic stem cell transplantation. LC-MS/MS is also used in endocrinology, where it has superior performance and sensitivity at low concentrations for many sex steroids. It also has applications in proteomics, where larger proteins or peptides can be digested before measurement. Immunoglobulins, which are key biomarkers for immunity, autoimmunity, cancer detection, and immune system function, can be overcome by LC-MS/MS methods.

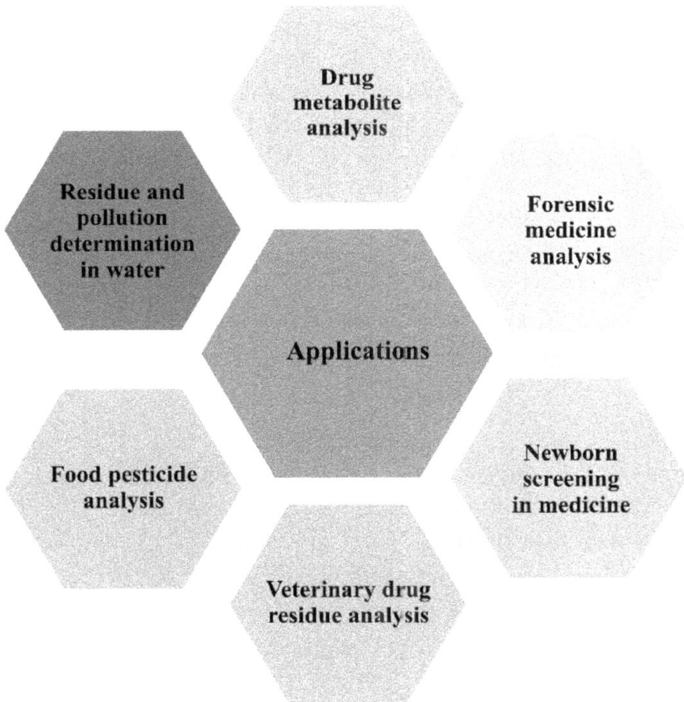

- **Used in quantification method for biogenic amines:**

  Neuroendocrine tumour identification requires the presence of naturally occurring substrates such as histamine, serotonin, and catecholamines, which are found in amines that are biogenic. Due to its increasing sensitivity and specificity, HPLC linked tandem mass spectrometry (LC-MS/MS) is quickly becoming a necessary technology in clinical chemistry laboratories. When it comes to identifying endocrine system abnormalities, this technique is very helpful in identifying biogenic amines, steroids, thyroid gland hormones, and vitamin D deficiency. Advanced sample pretreatment methods and process management are made possible by LC-MS/MS. Because of its increased specificity, faster runtimes, and easier sample preparation, it is frequently used in place of more traditional HPLC, GC-MS, and diagnostic procedures. Like HPLC and GC-MS, LC-MS/MS also permits the simultaneous detection of several substances.

- Used in therapeutic immunosuppressant's drug monitoring
- **Used in doping control:**

  In contemporary sports drug testing, LC-MS/MS has emerged as an essential element that supplements immunological and GC-MS(/MS)-based techniques for illicit substance detection. Utilizing high resolution/high accuracy MS, it provides quick, sensitive targeted analysis as well as untargeted screening processes. LC-MS/MS is now the go-to technique for quick, reliable, sensitive, and targeted detection in doping prevention labs. Although GC-MS was originally better at routine doping controls, LC-MS's capacity to identify a wide range of analytes at meaningful concentration levels has made it an indispensable tool. Though LC-MS/MS is more susceptible to ion suppression and matrix effects than GC-MS/MS techniques, it still has to contend with issues including both positive and adverse ionization, the production of multiple charged ions, and sufficient identification criteria.

References

1. Srividya Kailasam, LC-MS – What Is LC-MS, LC-MS Analysis and LC-MS/MS, Technology Networks analysis and separation, May 17, 2021, Last Updated: May 9, 2022.
2. https://www.slideshare.net/SantoshGandhi7/hplc-234926762
3. Paul Jannetto, Liquid Chromatography Tandem Mass spectroscopy, The Swiss Army Knife for Clinical Laboratories.

Questions

1. Write the principle, advantages and disadvantages of LC-MS/MS.
2. Add a note on instrumentation and applications of LC-MS/MS.
3. Write about mass analyzers with neat labelled diagram.

CHAPTER 15

Gas Chromatography Tandem Mass Spectrometer (GC-MS/MS)

Introduction

A single device called a tandem mass spectrometer uses two or more mass analyzers. The most basic configuration consists of two mass spectrometers (MS/MS) linked in series by a space called a collision cell. In essence, the material to be analyzed is sorted and weighed in the first mass spectrometer, broken into pieces in the collision cell, and then sorted and weighed in the second mass spectrometer. A collision cell separates each quadrupole in the tandem mass spectrometer, which is made up of two or more quadrupoles.

After chromatography has been used to separate a sample, the components first travel through an initial quadrupole, which separates the ion mixture and allowing specific ions (precursor ions) to pass through to the collision cell. The first quadrupole selects user-specified sample ions from a particular interest. These ions, called "parent ions," are bombarded with an inert gas and broken down into charged and mass ions (product ions). This procedure repeated numerous times to obtain results that are incredibly precise. The product ions, also known as "daughter ions," are used to separate ions and track specific ion pieces. Tandem mass spectrometers are utilized in various fields such as clinical investigations, toxicological studies, inborn metabolic defects, cancer, diabetes, toxins, and abuse-inducing substances. They are also used to identify pharmaceutical chemical makeup, detect contaminants, and locate medications in biological fluids and tissues.

Similar to GC-MS, GC-MS/MS requires materials to be separated using gas phase chromatography before being analyzed by a mass spectrometer. However, the tandem mass spectrometer employed in GC-MS/MS enables us to choose certain analytes for separate fragmentation. This makes it easier to analyze combinations that are more complicated.

The GC-MS/MS mass spectrometer employs an electron beam to ionize the analytes, but it also features a mode in which the electrons ionize an intermediary gas, which subsequently ionizes the analyte in secondary reactions. By minimizing the analytes' breakdown during ionization, this method enables more delicate fragmentation throughout the MS/MS phases.

Principle: GC-MS/MS analyses samples in a gaseous state and separates them based on the numerous physical and chemical characteristics of the target analytes and their interactions with the stationary phase of the analytical column. The analytes enter the tandem mass spectrometer (MS/MS), which is made up of two scanning mass analyzers separated by a collision cell, after leaving the analytical column. In the collision cell, fragments picked in the first analyser interact with an inert gas to fragment even further. The third quadrupole is then used to resolve these daughter product ions for analysis.

Instrumentation:

The components of GC-MS/MS are:

1. Gas chromatography
2. Mass spectrometer

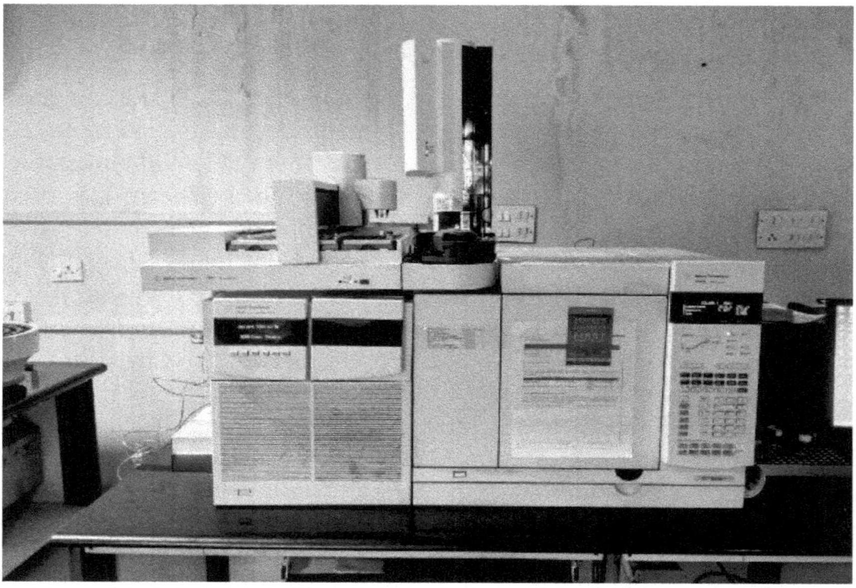

Fig.15.1 Instrumentation of GC-MS/MS.
https://images.app.goo.gl/RHpei6G3pKhHCW7MA

1. Gas chromatography:

I. Carrier Gas:

The carrier gas used in a sample depends on its composition, purity, accessibility, consumption, column efficiency, and detector type. Most commonly used are hydrogen, helium, nitrogen, argon. Helium is preferred due to its higher thermal conductivity, and its high pressure supply is monitored by pressure regulators and flow meters, affecting column efficiency.

Free-standing gas cylinders must be clamped to a support, and waste gases, particularly hydrogen, must be evacuated through an extraction cover. Numerous gases, such as air, hydrogen, and nitrogen, are accessible via benchtop generators that deliver high-purity gases at flow rates of 300 to 500 cm3 min due to safety concerns.

II. Sample injector:

Various devices are used to introduce liquid samples, such as a heated metal block injected with the sample using a hypodermic needle and a self-sealing silicone rubber septum, ensuring the sample port's temperature allows quick liquid evaporation without decomposition.

Split injection, splitless injection, direct on-column technique, thermal desorption, and pyrolysis are the injection systems now in use.

Split injection technique: Here, a heated injection port lined with glass is used to inject a 0.1 to 1.0 μl sample, which vapourizes and mixes with the carrier gas. Typically, only 1% to 10% of the sample is allowed to enter the column while the remainder is evacuated to the atmosphere using a variable needle valve. System prevents overloading issues by preventing carrier gas from being continually vented to the lab.

Splitless injection technique: However, this technology only works when material concentrations in the sample are high. The injector is used with a diluted solution in the volatile solvent, and the column temperature is adjusted to 293 K below the solvent's boiling point. The solvent trapping mechanism causes a plug of solvent to condense in the column, where it is concentrated by sample molecules. The split vent is opened 40 seconds later to remove solvent and prevent tailing and widening of peaks in the injector. Data acquisition depends on timing events and temperature in each stage of the technique. The solvent and low-boiling solute molecules are eluted quickly as a big peak. Separation can be successful if solute molecules have boiling temperatures 373-423 K higher than the solvent's boiling point.

Direct on-column Method for Sample Introduction: The maximum material handling capacity for a 0-25 mm column without overloading is 20 ng per component, equivalent to 0.005-0.05 liters of pure liquid. The syringe needle must be smaller than the column's internal diameter. Specialized pneumatic injection ports allow needle insertion directly onto the column head without obstructing carrier gas flow.

III. Oven:

Chemicals with varying boiling temperatures. Linear and non-linear temperature programming options are available for sample and reference columns. Vapour jackets or liquid baths can maintain column temperature at around 273.1K, ensuring consistent results.

IV. Column:

The column separation process involves analyzing the solid support, liquid phase type and quantity, packing method, column length, and temperature. A constant thermostat in an oven ensures predictable conditions, but the working temperature may vary from ambient to above 673 K.

Columns are of 2 types:

Packed columns: Glass, aluminum, copper, stainless steel, or high-temperature plastic are used to make packed columns. The columns are filled with graded adsorbent for GSC. The packing for GLC is made by covering an inert solid support with the liquid phase. Liquid phases can be either polar (carbowaxes) or non-polar (nujol, silicone gum rubber) or hydrogen-bonded glycol or glycerol.

Capillary columns: They depend on interaction between the stationary phase, which is deposited as a thin coherent film on the inner surface of a capillary tube, and the mixture. Fused silica, nylon, glass, copper, and stainless steel were employed in their construction. The capillary columns can be either packed (micropacked) or open tubular (with an open, unrestricted flow channel through the centre). Micropacked capillary columns have solid particles covering the whole diameter of the column.

In the latter, there are three types of columns: porous-layer open tubular (PLOT), support coated open tubular (SCOT), and wall coated open tubular (WCOT).

2. Mass spectrometer:

The most often used method is electron ionization, a higher energy method that can fragment the analyte species to help with structural clarification or offer confirming ions for quantitative measurement.

Ion-trap equipment, also known as tandem in time, has been used in MS-MS spectrum investigations for a long time. These instruments produce focused data for structural elucidation but have poor mass accuracy and resolution.

Due to high sensitivity, mass accuracy, and resolution requirements, most contemporary GC-MS-MS applications use "tandem in space" techniques.

The triple-quadrupole (QqQ) and quadrupole-time-of-flight (QTOF) combinations are commonly used commercially.

The orbital trap Fourier transform mass analyzer is a notable exception with extremely high resolution.

Triple quadrupole mass analyzer:

Designers connect three quadrupoles in series, the first and third of which are mass filters and each of which functions as a single quadrupole in a triple quad system. The samples are broken up by the center quadrupole using a collision gas, allowing for quantification of components or structural examination of samples.

SRM involves two steps of mass selection: selecting the mass of the intact targeted analyte (precursor ion) in the first quadrupole (Q1) and choosing a desired fragment (product ion) in the third quadrupole (Q3) following fragmentation of the Q1 mass-selected precursor ion by collision-induced dissociation in the second quadrupole (Q2). The desired fragment is then delivered to the detector, which records quantitative measurements based on the intensity profile of each transition. This process achieves high selectivity against co-cluting interferences, ensuring accurate measurements of the specific pair of precursor and product ions.

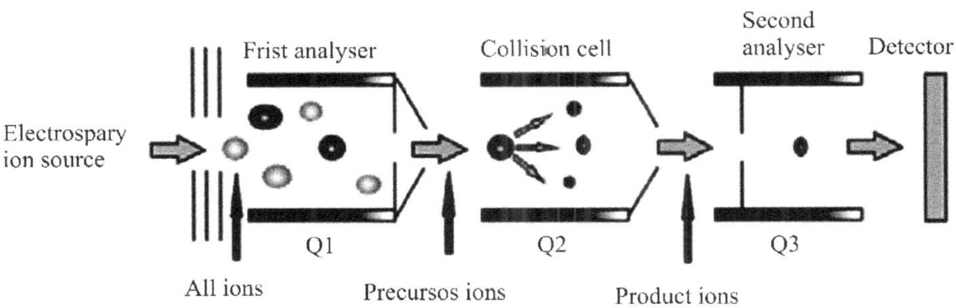

Fig.15.2 Triple quadrupole.
https://images.app.goo.gl/3SXYrHjp4UbU7wTq9

Quadrupole –TOF:

The Q-TOF-MS is a hybrid device that combines quadrupole technology with a time-of-flight mass analyzer. It is similar to a triple-quadrupole mass spectrometer, with the first quadrupole (Q1) serving as a mass filter and the second quadrupole (Q2) acting as a collision cell. The Q1 can be used in radio frequency (RF) alone mode to broadcast all ions, while the Q2 can operate in RF-only mode without ion fragmentation. The device is similar to a triple-quadrupole mass spectrometer.

Ions exit the quadrupole and enter the time-of-flight analyzer's ion modulator section, where they are accelerated by an electric field. They reach the flight tube, where mass separation occurs. Ions with lower mass travel farther and faster. Modern time-of-flight analyzers use a reflectron device to adjust for spatial spread and kinetic energy dispersion of ions with the same m/z but different velocities.

The Q-TOF-MS detector uses reflectron adjustment to allow ions with the same m/z to enter simultaneously, enhancing mass resolution. It uses quadrupole technology and a time-of-flight analyzer to perform two types of scans for data collection. In the first mode, unfragmented precursor ions are accurately mass scanned using the first and second quadrupoles in RF-only mode. A single mass or range of masses can be chosen for transmission to the TOF analyzer using the Q1. In the second mode, ions are sent into the collision cell (Q2) for CID.

The TOF analyzer accurately quantifies the mass of product and unbroken precursor ions, while the Q-TOF-MS can simultaneously gather information on both ions by switching between modes. A time-to-digital converter is used to convert ion flight time into a mass signal.

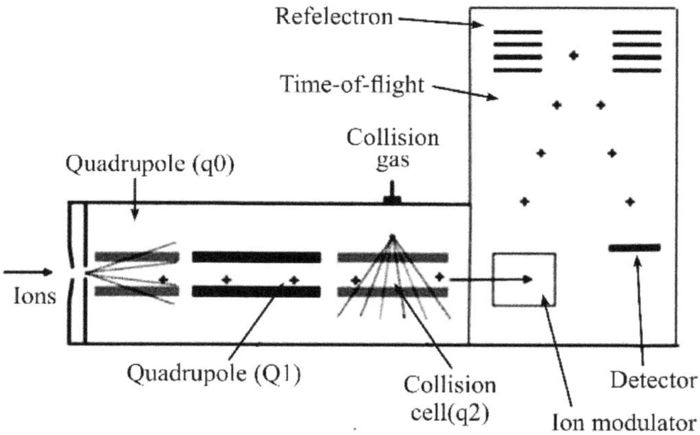

Fig.15.3 Quadrupole -TOF.
https://images.app.goo.gl/GndWxHo48hdXhvLm9

Advantages:

- GC-MS/MS may be used for quantitative processes by comparing signals to standards.
- It can also be utilized for the identification of volatile organic substances because of its high sensitivity EI source, ultimate sensitivity and selectivity, and large mass range up to 1050 m/z.
- It is very helpful for analyzing organic chemical traces.

Disadvantages:

- This technique is useful only for volatile compounds.
- The sample must undergo derivatization before analysis.

Applications:

1. **Environmental surveillance**:
   - Environmental pollution analysis and monitoring.
2. **Food safety:**
   - Food additive, food residue, contaminant, and unlawful additive detection.
3. **Biomedicine**:
   - Analysis of synthetic pharmaceuticals, synthetic APIs, and natural medications.
   - Analysis of tiny molecules, such as co-factors and amino acids, found in serum or urine.
   - In formulation science, chemical binders are analyzed.
4. **Legal science and toxicology:**
   - Analysis of poison and illicit substance.
5. **Phytochemistry**:
   - GC-MS/MS provides reliable identification and detection of phytoconstituents present in a plant extract
   - Used in identifying compounds include fatty acids, fatty alcohol, carboxylic acid, ion-chain alkanes, diterpenes, triterpenes, sterols and anthraquinones.

References

1. GCMSMS – 3500, Analytical Technologies Limited
2. Gas Chromatography Tandem Mass Spectrometry (GC-MS/MS); EAG laboratories
3. Gas Chromatography-Tandem Mass Spectrometry; JBL science
4. Shridhar Gawade, Basics of GC & GC-MS/MS and its applications in Food Safety, Thermo fisher scientific
5. H.Kaur, Instrumetal Methods of Chemical Analysis (Analytical Chemistry),Pragathi Prakashan
6. Ronald E Majors; M New chromatographic columns and accessories; LCGC North American; Volume-32, Issue-5

7. Darren R Allen and Brett C McWhinney, Quadrupole Time-of-Flight Mass Spectrometry: A Paradigm Shift in Toxicology Screening Applications, 2019 Aug; 40(3): 135–146.

Questions

1. What is meant by tandem spectroscopy?
2. List the applications of GC-MS/MS.
3. Write a note on GC-MS/MS.
4. Discuss about Quadrupole –TOF working.
5. Write a note on mass spectrometers.

www.ingramcontent.com/pod-product-compliance
Ingram Content Group UK Ltd.
Pitfield, Milton Keynes, MK11 3LW, UK
UKHW020047200726
13845UKWH00044B/11

9 789348 734426